Nobody's Listening to Me—
If Only They Could C Me:
A Daughter's Battle With Sickle Cell

Written By: Iris Wright-Hart
Illustrations By: Omani Valentin

Nobody's Listening to Me—If Only They Could C Me: A Daughter's Battle With Sickle Cell

Written By: Iris Wright-Hart
Illustrations By: Omani Valentin
Edited By: Aaron C. Butler

ISBN: 9781967082506 (Paperback)
ISBN: 9781967082513 (eBook)

Library of Congress Control Number: 2025918711

Printed in the United States of America

BookButler Publishing Company
Upper Marlboro, MD 20774

TheBookButler.com

BookButler Publishing Company titles may be purchased in bulk for educational, business, fundraising, or sales promotional use. For information, please email: info@thebookbutler.com

BookButler
PUBLISHING COMPANY

Dedication

FOR MY READERS

I hope the metaphors used in this book will give you visual insight into the impact of Sickle Cell.

Additionally, I am grateful for the feedback and interviews I have received from my husband, children, grandchildren, parents, siblings, closest relatives, friends, community and Sickle Cell Warriors who have inspired me to write.

A Message to All Who
Will Listen

We only see the outcome of it all, death. We are blind to the vision of it all. We are blind to looking in someone's eyes who is crying out in pain. We are blind to knowing they are sick and tired of being sick and tired. We are blind to the darkness they see day and night. We are blind when no one is listening to them about how they are feeling. We are blind to the many blood transfusions and blood exchanges that they are going through. We are blind to all the medications that are being pushed through their veins. We are blind to them, not knowing who they are, who they want to be, or who they can become. We are blind to them not being able to participate in all facets of life and enjoyment. We are blind to them dying from infancy to 52 years of age. We are blind to them, not knowing if they are going to live another day. We are blind to them fighting for their lives with every ounce of breath that remains in them.

Our vision should be the beginning of the future. Our beginning is at birth. I want my readers to know that you are responsible if you have inherited the trait from just one parent. This call to action is very imperative. If they have it, it means you have the trait for Sickle Cell Disease. When this happens, you are a Carrier. If we want to ensure the future of our generations, then we should consider getting tested before becoming a parent. All lives matter only when we can see the true vision of it all. Yes, all lives matter when we can see that this National and global disease is knocking at a lot of people's front doors because of the integration of cultures. Investigate your family's bloodline and health history.

Are you a future protagonist, one who advocates or is a champion of a particular cause or idea, one who is driven to action? Are you one who has a different point of view than one who presents background information? Authoring a book can cause you to find out things you didn't know. It can lead you down a path that is wide or narrow. I have discovered that whether having a conversation with people in a group or having a single conversation with one person, it seems to me that the majority of people have little to no knowledge of the disease itself, and even misconceptions. That would include me. I delve into extensive information on the nature and history of Sickle Cell from its Origins, the timeline, important dates in History, milestones, causes, research, treatment, and cures.

My insides are making me feel like shedding so many tears. The more I progress with writing this book, the harder it gets. It's like a roaring sea with the waves crashing down on me. It hurts, and I'm drowning along with my daughter. I want the beauty of a waterfall to make me rejoice with grace. Sometimes I feel my heart being inspired by the quiet morning glory, quiet afternoon delight, or the quiet of the night as I move forward in writing this book. Thoughts come rolling out of my mind so quickly that I am unable to contain them. My husband would say you write things down on everything or anything. I have to agree with him there, then I go on a scavenger hunt trying to find the thoughts of my writing on some inanimate object. That can be truly frustrating and a waste of time.

Sometimes I fear that my oldest girl, Mia, will never understand the love I have in my heart for her. Her heart has turned to stone in so many ways because of this infestation of Sickle Cell that causes her to become two different people. It has caused our relationship and those around her to laugh with her, cry with her, put up with her, stay away from her, become downhearted with her, rejoice with her, lose battles with her, and fight with her or for her. She is like a light switch, on and off.

In my opinion, that truly explains a lot of people who deal with Sickle Cell Crises. They are just sick of being tired and in pain. Many feel that no one is listening or seeing them. They put up a fight for their rights as a person and a patient. This chapter book is based on true-life stories and facts. I hope that I may not offend anyone with the facts that I have gathered from various resources, interviews, or quotes from other people, which I have found to be greatly beneficial. I hope that the songs and lyrics from songwriters, as well as the poetry from poets, will reach the hearts and souls, as well as the metaphorical expressions. Some of the names have been changed. I have included historical information about the names in my writings for this book because, for some, this is how people will be remembered from generation to generation. Some names talk about a person's reputation. Sometimes it can be the feelings of their parents at the time of the child's birth. May this book bring a sense of joy, laughter, calmness, enlightenment, and, above all, love for others. May the sounds of melodies ease the pain, anxiety, stress, and shame. May all uttered words heighten the reader's gratitude towards enlightenment valued in human happiness. A big shout-out goes to the Inspiration and Advocacy of the Sickle Cell Warriors.

Love Message

Love you, my daughter, Mia, which means mine. Ocean Goddess or Queen; also means "guardian of justice. That would be my Mia all the way. What a perfect name. It also means Moon (Australian origin that stems from the Noongar language of the Aboriginal people). My daughter admires the moon so much. She wears a moon necklace upon her neck every day for strength and guidance.

Much Love to My First-Born Child and First-Born Daughter. May you cherish my writings in this book forever.

FIGHT THE FINE FIGHT

SICKLE CELL WARRIORS

Table of Contents

Chapter 1

What's Happening to Me?
(Venomous Snake)

S nake Bite — Being bitten by a snake signals sudden danger and physical breakdown. Venom is now spreading, attacking tissue, swelling limbs, and destroying blood cells. A physiological fear, sweating, and shaking begin. The world begins to spiral, and control slips away. And with it comes pain — sharp, relentless, and alive in every breath.

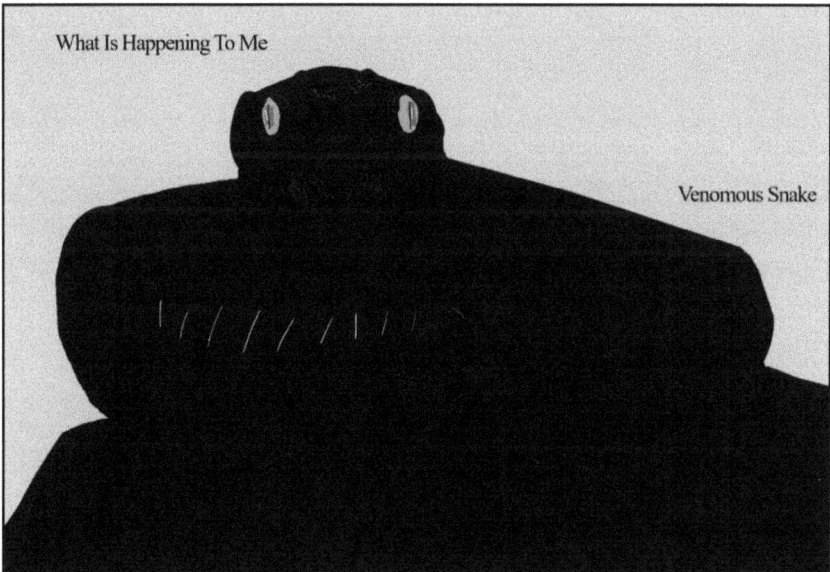

What Is Happening To Me

Venomous Snake

The Strike

Suddenly, Mena woke up in agony, as if someone had slammed a fist into her chest while she slept. The pain didn't stop there. It spread fast and wild, shooting through her arms, shoulders, legs, jaws, and back like sparks from a fire. Mena remembered reading about cobra snake bites in Science class and the effects of the venom. She felt like she had been bitten by a poisonous snake with its venom running throughout her body. Her hands were swelling, looking puffy and shiny. Her body pulsed with stabbing, throbbing pain — sharp and unrelenting, everywhere at once. Something was wrong. Terribly wrong.

Her body felt like it was unraveling. She couldn't explain it — only that each second brought a new wave of pain, deeper and more intense than the last. She was only fourteen. Weren't these supposed to be the fun years? The years of sleepovers and parties, of getting her first real crush? Not this.

If these are growing pains, she thought, *I don't want to grow anymore.* She clutched her sides and whispered aloud, "What on earth is happening to me?"

Lisa, her mom, had talked to her about what to expect. When certain changes came, her body shifted into something new. But this…wasn't that. This was something ancient and punishing. It felt like being stretched on a torture rack, like those stories from history class where prisoners were pulled until their bodies begged for mercy. That's what her body was doing now: begging. And it was losing. The pain was unbearable, excruciating.

Yesterday, the Beach

It was a cold, rainy day that showed no mercy to Mena. The sun seemed to be playing hide and seek, offering her no warmth at all. Just yesterday, things had been different. At the beach with her friends and family, Mena's body had soaked up the radiant warmth of the sun. Mena remembered running vigorously in the hot sand. The sand was flying up behind her heels. Her legs felt as though she had just finished track practice — or run a full marathon. She sat on the sand, hoping she wouldn't wake up sore, with pain coursing through her body the next day.

Now the effect of her running hard had snuck up on her. The pain was running through her body like waves crashing down on her. It felt like her pain was taking on a life of its own, ruling how she was feeling, thinking, and breathing. It was the most insufferable level of pain you could imagine. Mena thought for a moment, second-guessing herself about the agony of the pain she was having. She knew that her mother would wholeheartedly disagree with that statement.

Her mother always said that childbirth was the most painful thing you could ever go through. It is the closest a woman could get to death.

Gasping, Mena said, "This pain… It's up there with childbirth. I know it is."

The Cry for Help

She felt herself gasping for air, as if her oxygen were slipping away. The pain struck everywhere — sudden, sharp, and unpredictable. It gripped her chest, twisted through her abdomen, and pulsed in waves she couldn't escape.

Mena screamed at the top of her voice, "Mommy… Mommy, it hurts! My chest— I can't move— everything hurts!"

Tears poured down her face.

Lisa began to panic! What could be wrong with her child?

Lisa got lost in a memory, thinking about the chest pain she sometimes felt — the kind that left her frozen, unable to move. "No. It can't be the same thing…can it?" Lisa recognized that pain. She had felt it herself: crushing… breath-stealing… impossible to ignore. But she had never seen it in Mena, until now.

Lisa pushed the thought aside — there was no time to dwell. She had to act. Mena had managed to scream, and that alone was a miracle. Her cry tore through the house, raw and desperate — the kind of sound that made you wonder if someone was dying. Was she? Lisa's heart raced as she pulled Mena into her arms and shouted for her husband.

"What is it? What's wrong?" Bruce said with a strained voice as he rushed into the room.

Lisa turned to her husband, her voice shaking, "We have to get Mena to the hospital — now. Look at her, she's in so much pain and doesn't even know why. We've gotta go. We've gotta go!"

There was no time to pack a bag. No time to think about who to call. Just a mother, a father, a child — and a fear racing faster than the car, desperate for answers.

Chapter 2

The Ride to the Hospital
(Waves of the Sea)

Waves are created by energy passing through water, causing it to move in a circular motion. Waves are most commonly caused by wind. The gravitational pull of the sun and moon on the Earth also causes waves. https://oceanservice.noaa.gov

Pain Rising

Waves build quietly, then crash without warning. That's how fear moves, too—steady, rising, unstoppable. On the way to the hospital, Mena could think of nothing more than the pain she was experiencing, and she just wanted it to stop. Mena's heart was racing. She was having shortness of breath. She was trying to think of a breathing technique that would help; however, she could barely think. Mena's body was beginning to tremble out of control. She felt her legs weakening from all the tension that was going on within her body. It was like a weight that no one would ever want to bear. The pain was all-consuming. But a question kept pulsing through her mind: Is this the end of my teenage years? She didn't know if she believed in God, but right now she hoped someone was listening. If there was ever a need for prayer, now would be the time. She did feel as if there was a higher power, and her mother's prayer would do for now. If it would help, then so be it. Her grandmother, WaWa, would always say that when she knew that nothing would change. She knew that her parents were going to take care of that part of her life, prayer – if necessary.

The Hammer and the Memory

Mena described the pain as someone using a hammer against her body like a baseboard. To distract her, she thought about her uncle's Roadkill hammer stories. The way he could build anything. What a strange name for a man. He got that name because people would tease him about picking up animals that had been hit by a car. They often thought of him taking it home and cooking the roadkill on the road. He ate and cooked so many strange things like turtle pie, deer, squirrels, muskrats, and the list could go on with his wild animal eating. He was very industrious as well. Mena remembered when he would tell her stories about when he was a little boy.

One of his stories was about his brother, Road Racer, and his friends. He called his brother Road Racer because he was always racing up and down the road with his cartwheel. Mena remembered her uncle telling her about how they would walk to the dump to find some boards and nails. On their way back home, they would meet up with their neighborhood friends so that they could help them build log cabins. They would hammer all day and sometimes throughout the night. That was exactly how Mena was feeling—like something was being hammered in her chest day and night. Mena thought some more about how her uncle is still building so many things today, like outdoor gyms for his grandchildren. They now have swings, monkey bars, and obstacles to run through. Mena could see the sweat protruding from his face, just like the tears that were profusely coming down her face. Throughout the memories of all his hammering, Mena's mind returned to thinking about the throbbing in her heart. Her uncle would hammer with all his might, as if he were a madman. She no longer wanted to think about her Uncle hammering anything. Mena knew that he could break anything or build anything. But this pounding? This wasn't something even he could fix.

Mena felt that she was too young for something to be wrong with her heart until today. Would the doctors prove her wrong?

Fractured Memories, Rising Fear

Another cry tore from Mena's throat, "Daddy, please make the pain stop. Are we almost there?"

Bruce flinched at the sound of her scream. He hadn't heard pain like that in years—not since his college days, when a frat brother's howl during pledge week haunted him for months. Bruce got branded on his chest. He remembered the clinching of his teeth, trying not to make a sound. That's what Mena was trying to do: not make a sound. Bruce knew that his frat brother had screamed so loudly that his painful outburst frightened even him. But this? This was his daughter. And he was helpless.

Inside the Car, Inside the Chaos

Bruce had driven as if he were on a speed track, racing in and out of lanes. He was putting the pedal to the metal in a race for his daughter's survival, her life, or so he thought. The adrenaline in his body was rising higher and higher with every mile. He felt his blood pressure rising with every scream of pain coming from his daughter. His heartbeat was racing with all the anxieties of life coming down upon him. His temperature was rising so quickly that he could now feel tingling in his legs. He remembered the way his legs would feel when he traveled for hours in a car. When that happened, Bruce would always stop at a visitors' center for a break to walk around. However, he knew that this was not possible to do. Bruce had to keep driving no matter what. He was beginning to wonder if he would survive this ordeal himself.

Lisa was terrified as the passenger, for she had been diagnosed with vertigo, so she was busy panting and taking deep breaths. It felt like how the Bible describes being tossed about like a ship on the sea, carried here and there by every kind of wind. Mena felt like a surging wave that was engulfing all her anxieties. Lisa knew that she had to conquer those waves she was feeling. She could not let these waves of anxiety prevail. Lisa knew she had to pull herself together by using her taught techniques of breathing and counting.

Arrival

This was one of the times that Lisa could feel the oneness of her husband and herself. Lisa was sure he was feeling the same emotions she was feeling. Lisa was feeling waves of anxiety with no beginning or end. All sorts of emotions were upon them both. Flash Floods of thoughts surrounding them every second, minute, of time. Bruce parked at the emergency entrance and opened his car door. Finally, they had reached their destination, the hospital. Lisa never could have imagined the hospital grounds being a beautiful sight. It had roses, geraniums, and daffodils all around the walkways. However, nothing was more beautiful than the gray metal doors of the hospital. Mena leaps into his arms. The doors slid open, and Bruce didn't wait. He rushed inside. "Help! Please—someone help us!"

Desperate Words

Upon entering the hospital, a nurse rushed toward them with a wheelchair. Bruce lowered Mena in as gently as he could, but she let out a cry as her body shifted. Lisa was already at her side, trying to explain…

"She—woke up screaming—said it felt like a fist in her chest, like somebody hit her while she was sleeping—she kept saying it was like a hammer, like her body was being nailed to something–her hands were swell, she couldn't move—she said everything hurt, her chest, her legs, her jaw —everywhere! She was gasping, like the air wouldn't come—she said it felt like waves, like she was drowning in it, like something ancient, like she was being torn apart—please, please, just help her!"

The nurse didn't hesitate. Mena was wheeled straight through the doors.

Bruce staggered toward the front desk to check her in, hands shaking as he fumbled for his wallet. Lisa followed the wheelchair, her daughter's words echoing in her head: "Mommy, my chest is hurting me and my whole body. I can't move."

First Diagnosis

After all was said and done, the doctor came back with the nightmare news. "The blood test results have come back. Lisa has a genetic blood disorder where her red blood cells are not the normal disc shape. These abnormal shapes are blocking the blood flow. It is causing her severe pain in various parts of her body, shortness of breath, and can cause organ damage. We have taken several types of blood tests, and your daughter has been diagnosed with Sickle Cell Anemia."

Lisa collapsed into the nearest chair, sobbing. The words echoed in her ears—Sickle Cell. She was overwhelmed by the news. She knew what that meant.

Pain. Hospitals. Fear. Maybe worse.

How long would Mena have to suffer?

How long before…before she—

Lisa couldn't finish the thought. She looked at Bruce, eyes wide. Neither of them had answers. Only the doctor could tell them what came next.

"We'd like to transfer her to Johns Hopkins. They'll be able to give her more specialized care."

So they went—still shaken, still unsure.

A Different Name

When all the blood tests were taken at Johns Hopkins, the doctor came into the room and said, "She doesn't have Sickle Cell Anemia, which people call Sickle Cell Disease (SS). She has a form of Sickle Cell Anemia. She has Hemoglobin Sickle Cell, which is called HbSC. They both cause pain episodes and a type of anemia. HbSC is usually a much milder form. Anemia is when the red blood cells break down faster than they should. She can also experience tiredness or weakness."

Lisa said to the doctor, "Can you simplify what you are saying?"

The doctor said, it's a genetic disorder where your daughter has inherited one gene for sickle cell hemoglobin (S) and one for hemoglobin (C). She has inherited Heterozygous. The doctor saw the look on their confused faces. He said, "It means Mena has inherited one abnormal gene and one normal gene. One from each parent. We will give you a pamphlet, where it will be broken down so that you can understand what I am saying much better."

The Long Road Ahead

"Will she be in pain like a person with Sickle Cell or die at a young age?" Lisa asked.

The doctor replied, "Generally, HbSC(Hemoglobin Sickle Cell) has less severe symptoms than are associated with HbSS(Hemoglobin Sickle Cell Anemia). I do know that her complications with HbSC can cause her pain, fatigue, anemia, and splenomegaly. It can also mess with her sight. It's called retinopathy. She may develop Avascular Necrosis."

Bruce said, "What's that?"

The doctor replied, "It's the death of bone tissue. That's due to a lack of blood supply to the bone. Later, I will refer your daughter to a hematologist to discuss the treatment options for HbSC. I can say that it will include medication, antibiotics, therapies, and possibly blood transfusions."

Out of the Storm—for Now

Bruce and Lisa were relieved to know that the diagnosis given by their home hospital was incorrect. They knew that their daughter was not out of the woods. They also knew this was going to take a lot of prayer. They would have to be by their daughter's side for the long journey she was about to undertake.

Lisa felt that they were in a whirlwind of words they couldn't understand. A situation that was going at a fast pace. Everything that they had been experiencing was developing so quickly. Lisa and Bruce felt as if their world was being turned upside down. Mena's life and their life were headed for a rough sea. Lisa and Bruce felt just like the Psalm of David. *"Their strength evaporated like water in the dry summer heat."* They could bear no more for the day.

Chapter 3

Beyond the Pain of Sickle Cell (Childbirth)

Childbirth is the process of delivering a baby. Labor and delivery describe the process of childbirth. Contractions of the uterus and changes in the cervix (opening of the uterus) prepare a woman's body to give birth. Then the baby is born, and the placenta follows. There are 4 types of childbirth: Vaginal delivery, Assisted vaginal delivery (vacuum or forceps), C-section, and VBAC (Vaginal birth after cesarean). https://www.nichd.nih.gov

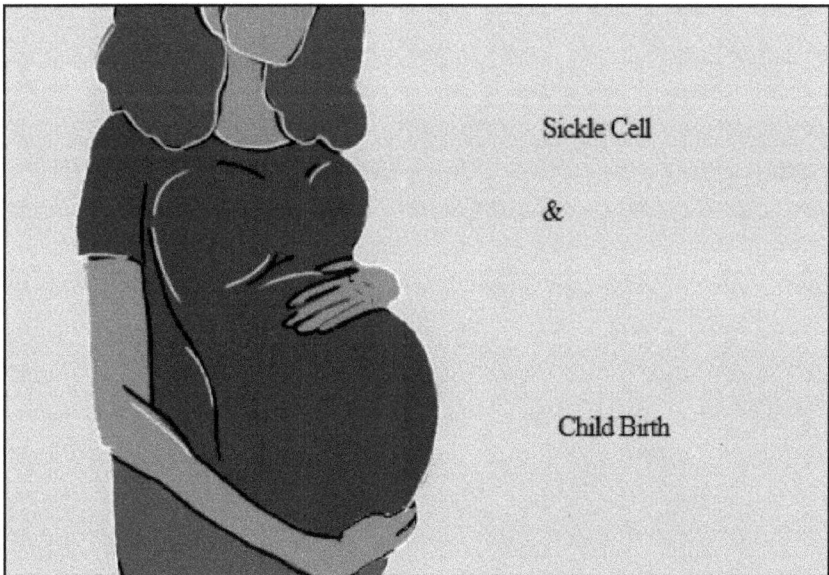

Sickle Cell

&

Child Birth

Mena vs. Lisa's experience of Giving Birth Experience

Mena was a vaginal delivery; however, with the children Mena gave birth to, she was able to experience all 4 types of childbirth. Mena took her time coming into this world. Lisa was in labor for twelve hours. The pain was something Lisa never wanted to go through ever again. Lisa was extremely fortunate to never have discomfort in her back with pain; however, the abdominal pain was out of this world. How could anyone survive this pain? Lisa had never experienced menstrual cramps, so this, this right here, was unimaginable. Lisa knew when it was almost time for Mena, her unborn child, to come because she would just be walking along, and all of a sudden, a strange shot of pain would hit her pelvic area, and she was unable to walk. The baby had dropped into her pelvis. This would be followed by lower abdominal pressure. She was constantly going to the bathroom all the time. The baby was pushing down on her bladder. The doctor said that it would be two or four weeks before she would most likely go into labor. Lisa was waiting for this day to come.

Doctor's Visits

During Lisa's doctor's visit, the doctor said that she had only dilated two centimeters. Lisa figured she had time before the baby came. She needed to dilate ten centimeters. Of course, every woman's time during labor pain is different. It's a gradual process for some, which can take up to two weeks; for others, it can last as long as a month, and for some, it can happen overnight, just like that. Lisa's husband often helped her get to where she was going or just assisted her in sitting in the chair. If any of this had happened to Mena, the doctor would have called for Mena to come in right away.

Natural Birth

The doctor did not want Mena to go into labor at the slightest. Mena's doctor had decided that she would not have a natural birth. He knew that if she did, there would be pain involved for her to have a baby naturally because of her Sickle Cell. It would cause Mena to go into a crisis. Mena would never experience natural childbirth, or her body telling her what time her firstborn child was coming. Mena's doctor had scheduled the time and the date for delivery because she could be at a higher risk for other complications. It's a known fact that most women who have Sickle Cell Disease need to be monitored closely during labor and delivery. Mena's doctor felt that she was a high risk, especially because of her history of having frequent crises. All the things that would be considered during Mena's delivery were Fetal monitoring, Hydration (giving fluids through an IV), Oxygen (Extra), and Postpartum monitoring (risk of blood clots). Mena's doctor wanted to avoid treating a crisis with intervention methods as well such as Blood transfusions, Blood exchanges, fluid replacement therapy, oxygen therapy, and steroids.

Lisa and her mom, Ann, had decided to go shopping. Ironically, Lisa's mom's name, Ann, means suffering from pain. That's exactly what was happening to Lisa. She was suffering from pain. Lisa often had to stop walking because of the pain in her legs. Lisa would take the time to take deep breaths.

Ann said, "Girl, you are about to have this baby soon, so we'd better cut our shopping short."

Later that evening, Lisa's mom decided to take a late nap.

Lisa walked into the room, "Mom, my stomach is hurting."

Lisa's Delivery

Ann replied, "Go and take some Pepto Bismol."

That didn't work, so Lisa returned to her mother's bedroom and said, "Mom, my stomach is hurting; the Pepto Bismol didn't work."

Mena's doctor, of course, would not have recommended Pepto Bismol. He would have found a safer way to treat the pain, such as changing Mena's medicine, which would be safe for her and the baby. He would have asked her to have someone give her a massage or use breathing techniques to help her relax.

Ann immediately jumped out of bed and said, "Girl, you are getting ready to have this baby."

This was not Braxton Hicks because the pain was not easing up, no matter what change of position Lisa put herself in. The pain was coming more frequently and more intensely. Sometimes the pain was less painful, and sometimes the pain lasted longer than others.

Ann said, "Oh my goodness, we've got to get you to the hospital."

Ann quickly got on the phone with Lisa's husband, Bruce, who was out of town on a job assignment. "Bruce, I am on my way to take Lisa to the hospital. She has gone into labor." Bruce didn't waste any time making a reply and said, "I will be there as soon as I can."

There were no phone calls for Mena when it was time for her to deliver her baby. The relationship Mena had with her baby's father was history. Mena and Keith had gone their separate ways.

Mena didn't hear those words come out of Keith's mouth: "I will be there as soon as I can." Like her father's words were to her mother

Mena didn't want him there anyway. Lisa's body had gone through so many changes before she went into labor. There were frequent contractions, cramps, diarrhea, weight gain, fatigue, and the waiting for her water to break. She was so excited, nervous, and anticipating this day to come. Twelve hours later, Lisa told the doctor the baby was coming.

The doctor said, "No, it's not time yet, you have only dilated 7 centimeters."

Lisa screamed, "I don't care what you think, the baby is coming. I can feel it."

The doctor decided to examine Lisa again. "Oh, my goodness," the doctor said, "the baby is coming." It's a girl. This was true happiness—Lisa's first baby.

Mena's Delivery Experience

Mena never heard those words from her doctor. Mena's delivery was a planned delivery. In Mena's case, the doctor used forceps to help move Mena's baby through the birth canal. Lisa thought the forceps looked like 2 large salad forks. The doctor had to guide the baby's head out of the birth canal. Lisa remembered what the baby's head looked like. It was the shape of a cone, and there were marks left on both sides of his head. The doctor kept telling Mena not to push because his sole purpose was for Mena not to go into a crisis.

He was the most caring doctor. He treated Mena as if she were his own. The atmosphere was so loving and caring. Mena loved the way the doctor cared mentally and physically—finally, a baby boy. Mena delivered vaginally with no pain. The doctor's method had worked. The doctor had kept her from going into a crisis. Mena had fallen in love with her brand-new baby boy. It wasn't long before Mena had postpartum depression after her delivery. Mena was having Baby Blues: negative feelings, sadness, and mood changes. In time, it turned into depression throughout her life.

The Naming of Mena

Bruce hadn't made it to the hospital yet because he was 5 hours away. He was having trouble getting there because his car had broken down on the mountainous highway. After walking for 2 miles, a stranger finally stopped for him as he was thumbing his way to get to the hospital. Bruce finally made it before the baby's arrival into the world. It's a girl! Lisa examined every inch of her precious daughter, making sure the hospital made no mistake of giving her the wrong baby when they would have to take her away for an examination and then return her baby to her.

Lisa told Bruce, "I want to name her Mena. It means mine. She is our baby."

Bruce agreed that it was a lovely name because his wife had been through so much for months, and that the reasoning behind the name meant something.

Lisa looked over at Bruce and said, "Honey, you look bad. What's wrong?"

Bruce said, "I have a fever. My car broke down, and I had to walk and hitchhike through the freezing weather. I'd better go home and take something and rest. Do you mind? Our daughter is beautiful. She is our little princess always. I will always love her forever, the way I will always love you from the heart."

Personality Change

Their precious, beautiful daughter grew up in so many ways. She was smart, strong, and lovable. As the years went by, Mena's pain turned her lovable ways into anger and hostility. Mena's lovable ways would surface occasionally. Every so often, she would be filled with love, joy, and laughter.

Lady Blackbird once sang, "Distance Turns to Blue, I'll Fix It for You." The day Lisa and Bruce found out that Mena had HbSC, they realized they could no longer correct it for Mena. Lisa was feeling the blues since Mena lived so far away, and Mena was feeling the same way. Mena felt as if she shouldn't care about a lot of things and that others didn't care either. The pain of not feeling loved was worse than the pain of childbirth. Labor pains were temporary. They come and go, and then the pain is soon forgotten. Your physical body goes through so many changes, and there is a cure for it. It's called time. Most of all, at the end of giving birth, you are so overwhelmed with joy that pain is only a distant memory in your mind. The feeling of not being loved can scare you for life. Mena had been through lots of things emotionally, and she felt as if the wound within her would never heal.

Mena thought, *"If God is a God of love, how can He allow any person to go through such an awful disease alone. No one knows how you truly feel inside or the pain that you are going through."*

My Best Isn't Good Enough

Mena's distance from her family had turned to feeling Blue. She had been experiencing cold, dreary, rainy days. Mena would take the pain of childbirth over the pain of heartbreak. Her Sickle Cell Crisis had caused a distance between her and her family, as well as anyone that she had tried to love.

Mena expressed to Lisa, "I feel as though I am constantly looked down upon. I feel that no matter what I do, it's never going to be good enough for anyone. I know you guys think that I am a failure because I haven't been able to accomplish the things that you both wanted so much for me. I had a child right out of high school, and I didn't finish college on your time. I'm not even the mother you expected me to be because you had to help me raise my child. My patience and tolerance were not there because pain seemed to follow me everywhere. I'm sure there has been a lot of talk behind my back among you guys and my family and friends. I once heard you say to April not to be like your sister. You don't want to end up like her. Well, at least in my mind, that's what I thought I heard you say. Am I such a bad person? My best isn't good enough. I figure the only way to be happy is to make myself happy. I've always worried about what you guys are thinking. Well, no more because it hurts too much when I don't succeed. I'm going to have a nervous breakdown at such an early age. The more pressure you put on a person who loves you, the harder they fall. I've fallen too many times. It's time for me to rise on my own. It's time for me to put my suicidal thoughts behind me, that I am not good enough."

Mena knew that she would never rise on her own without help, because this pain that she was having with Sickle Cell would always knock her to her feet, and she would always eventually come calling for her parents, family, and friends for support.

Love of a Child

Mena continued, "I wish things were different. You guys just make me feel bad. When I had my first child, I felt as if you guys didn't love me as much as I thought you loved Mario because he was young and new. You will see soon that things will be different. I know what you are thinking."

Lisa felt the pain of Mena's words echoing inside of her. Yes, Mena's emotional words were worse than the pain of Sickle Cell itself. It was bruising Lisa's heart. A cloud of sadness was creeping in on her, instead of a ray of sunshine.

Lisa replied, "You say I feel as if you're not good enough. Well, how could a child that has come out of my womb not be good enough? As I closed my eyes, I felt every movement of you, every kick, every hiccup, and every roll of you within me. I said to myself, 'This baby is truly a gift from God.' He saw your embryo from the beginning. So, I knew that you were a special part of me. I agree that I would never know the physical and mental pain that you are going through if I had never experienced it. I can only feel the pain that I see with my own eyes. The pain I see when my daughter is rolled up as an infant, as if she were still inside of me. When I see the outcry of your moaning and groaning, I moan and groan too because I can't make the pain go away that my child is feeling. I feel the pain of hopelessness. I hear the sound of unwelcome agony ripping through my ears. It transmits from one place to another within my soul, causing me pain and misery. I just stand there in silence with empty words of nothingness. As for the things that I wanted you to accomplish. I don't truly know. I only know that deep down inside, I only wanted you to be able to take care of yourself and not need any man to take care of you. I always knew that mother instinct would come the day you took Mario back. Giving birth to a child is never a forgotten thing. Your love for them will always remain inside you. You gave and are still giving all that you can, regardless of the constant fights you are having with your own body. Who could be stronger than someone who comes out on top with this horrid disease? I knew he would come first in your life. Everything else would go on the back burner. I remember the day you were scheduling and planning every moment for your child while you were in the hospital.

Sickle Cell pains will never compare with the Birth pains of a mother; the outcome of giving birth is called LOVE. The outcome of Sickle Cell is called death."

Beyond the Pain of Childbirth

Lisa realized that her daughter's pain was suffering beyond the pain of Sickle Cell. There was something more painful than Sickle Cell and childbirth. It was the pain resulting from not feeling loved. The emotional bond that they both wanted seemed as if it had disappeared into thin air, like the mist that fell upon the earth. They both were too busy to read between the lines. Life had truly gotten in the way. They were no longer expressing the feelings they had for one another as mother and daughter. The pain had conquered love. They were both blindsided by it. The temperament of motherhood resulting from the struggle with Sickle Cell had gotten in the way. They could never see eye to eye on most things that they used to share.

Lisa thought to herself, *"Where had my little girl gone? My pride and joy, my heart."*

Deep down, Lisa knew that Mena still loved her because whenever Mena was in a crisis —whether it was due to pain, doctors, nurses, family, or even her relationships with men —Mena would call and ask for her opinion. She just wanted her mom to make things right.

There were times when Mena would say, "I never want to speak to you again, or I don't need you, I got this!"

Lisa would feel pain in her heart, and as time passed by, Mena would forget her words and welcome Lisa back into her life. Pain can make you unsociable. There were times when Mena would lose her best friends because she just didn't care. Mena would be in a lonely place because her friends would just stop coming. They knew Mena's temperament and rage. Mena experienced headaches and fatigue often because of pain, so most of the time, she just wanted people to go away and leave her alone. The doctor once put her on medicine for depression, but Mena felt that it just made matters worse. She felt as if she had the energy of a sloth. Her mind was moving in slow motion. She was unable to get anything done around the house. She just wanted to sleep. She felt that way a lot every time she came from the hospital. She couldn't determine whether it was the exhaustion from the medicine's effect on her body, fighting with the doctors, or whether it was her body fighting from the Sickle Cell Crisis. Maybe it was pain from the crisis coming and going. Now, if you compare it to childbirth, the pain that you are going through pushing, stop pushing, pushing, stop pushing, almost took the life out of you. Mena just didn't know which one was worse. The older Mena got, the more she felt that she was getting more and more exhausted from all this fighting. The smallest task seemed so challenging to her. She could barely lift a finger at times. Mena was eating and sleeping too much or too little. She was pulling away from people and things. She was having low or no energy at all. The pain she was going through was unexplained aches and pains, such as constant stomach aches or headaches. Most of all, she was feeling helpless or hopeless.

Mena and Lisa had experienced all these emotions of distress, especially Mena. She was always fighting to try and find her way out. Mena felt as though she might need to go and see a psychiatrist or a mental health professional. She blames the way she was feeling on childbirth. Maybe having four kids was too many times. Maybe it was too much for someone who had HbSC. Anyone who has Sickle Cell has experienced all of these forms of emotional distress in one way or another if they have felt pain. Mena was determined that she was strong, and she would conquer all of this, especially the pain of not feeling loved.

Chapter 4

Desensitized Siblings (Roller Coaster)

Roller Coaster Attitude is a perspective or mindset that can influence how someone experiences a situation or event with sudden and extreme changes. For example, someone might describe a relationship as an emotional rollercoaster if it experiences periods of ups and downs. A situation or experience that alternates between making you feel excited, exhilarated, or happy and making you feel sad, disappointed, or desperate. This trip has been an emotional roller coaster for me. https://www.quora.com

Mena's life was truly full of ups and downs, with emotions starting at the age of thirteen. She would have many emotional highs and lows. She had no control over when her crisis would begin or end. Some days she was happy and excited about life, and some days she would feel sad and disappointed about the way her teenage years were going. Mena's crisis started coming more frequently. Mena's crisis came so often like a roller coaster. It had so many twists and turns that her siblings began to be desensitized. "They sometimes kept their distance, not knowing what version of Mena they'd get– joyful or overwhelmed by pain.

Chris Memories

Lisa remembered her son, Chris, becoming desensitized. He was no longer alarmed at the sight of Mena going to the hospital. Mena had come in and out of the hospital during her time when Chris was growing up. Come to think of it, Mena was twelve years older than her baby brother, Chris. When Mena started experiencing and going through her Sickle Cell Crisis, Chris was only five years old. He only remembered Mena going back and forth out of the house. It didn't seem to bother him much on all the trips Mena had been taking. He knew that Mena would come back the same day or someday soon. Chris felt that she would come back home and be all right. Psychologically, it just didn't bother him anymore. He wasn't aroused anymore by the ruckus that took place in the house, so he didn't pay much attention to her going to wherever it was anymore.

Lisa recalled asking Chris what he remembered about Mena when he was older, and Chris replied, jokingly, "I am getting my lawyer."

Lisa said, "But you don't have a lawyer."

Chris said, "If you have a phone, you have a lawyer."

Lisa replied, "So who might that be?"

Chris said, "Whoever I call at Saiontz & Kirk."

They both laughed at one another. They remembered the commercial by Saiontz & Kirk Attorneys saying, "If you have a phone, you have a lawyer. Chris always had jokes. Lisa also replied, "There is a Free Injury Hotline 7 Days/Nights. Hope you won't need one, silly boy." Lisa and Chris both laughed at each other again.

Lisa asked, "What else is it that you remember about your sister?"

Chris said, "Um, I just remember in Montana, the high altitude that it didn't work well with her Sickle Cell condition. I just remember it kind of seemed like once every other month, at least she'd be in the hospital for a little while, and it just became part of her life, just about. Like her being there because of her condition. Just the pain she would be in. The cramps and mostly pain."

Lisa remembered asking him if there was anything that he felt he could do.

Chris said, "I didn't feel like there was anything that I could do to help because I didn't understand it."

Chris only knew that the cell looked different from a normal cell and just the pain that it caused the body. He didn't know why it caused pain.

He only said, "I know that it looks like an instrument like a Sickle tool." Chris also said, "I know that Mena and her cousin, Autumn, had blood transfusions, at least I know Autumn has."

Lisa thought hard; she remembered even asking Chris, "Do you know why they had blood transfusions?

Chris's answer was "NO. I know their eyes well; at least Autumn's eyes are yellow."

Lisa said, "Yeah, Jaundice."

Chris took a deep breath and said, "I remember going to the hospital with her one time, and it was terrible. Mena was in a lot of pain, and it was a long wait in that waiting room. I don't remember what we talked about, but I just remember us talking." Chris took another deep breath, "I don't even remember having a conversation with any of the doctors or nurses. There were a lot of people just waiting in pain. Sorry, Mom, it was just so long ago. I don't remember a lot of things or how I was feeling. You have to remember that she was gone a lot when I was a kid. She had already moved out when I was in middle school. I wasn't around her a lot growing up. I just remember her in the hallway of our house singing, "Spiderwebs," which was funny."

Lisa laughed and repeated what Chris had said: "Spiderwebs song." Chris said, "Yeah, it was a song by Ahhh, No Doubt, the name of the Song was 'Spiderweb."

Lisa said, "Did you sing with her?"

Chris said, "Nuh, I just remember her singing that song. Like I said, our age difference was like 12 years. I also remember I was playing Nintendo when she went into labor, so that messed up my Super Mario Bros. Game."

Lisa said, "What?" And they both laughed together again, even though it wasn't a laughing matter. Chris raised his voice and said, "Because she had to go to the hospital. Everybody was rushing because she was about to give birth to Mario. People were just hustling and bustling. Running all around me. I thought I was going to be trampled on. That's all I remember."

"Oh, just one more thing, I also remember this cool boyfriend of hers, Juan, that I liked a lot because we used to play video games and watch wrestling together on the couch. He was a great memory in my life."

Chris thought that from the outside looking in, Juan was an impressive guy. He looked at him as being his friend.

"I was sad when he left."

Chris had heard his mom and Mena talking, and Mena was crying, and she said, "I thought he loved me."

Lisa bowed her head in sadness because she had liked him too. That's when she saw Mena for the first time, happy in a relationship. Lisa also remembered Chris telling her about a football player and a rapper.

Lisa remembered Chris saying, "There was this football player, Ryan Clark, who plays for the Pittsburgh Steelers, and they weren't sure if he was going to be able to play in Sunday's AFC Wild Card game in Denver because of the high altitude. It would make it dangerous. They didn't know how that would affect his Sickle Cell.

Lisa knew Chris had also told her about a rapper named Prodigy who died of complications related to his Sickle Cell Anemia.

Truth be told, Chris didn't know which one of his parents had the trait or if they both did. He knew most likely he or his sisters would have Sickle Cell or the trait. He had hoped that it wasn't him for either.

When Chris eventually got married, he wished that Mena had met his wife, Maria, under different circumstances. Maria was passionate, and she put her heart and soul into everything that her family and Chris's family did. Mena was going through a crisis when they first met, and Mena was not incredibly happy about seeing Maria at that moment for the first time. She wasn't even sure if she would like her because she wasn't black. Mena had friends of different nationalities, but she was prejudiced against some that she didn't know, especially if they were white. Maria was extremely nervous about meeting Mena as well because of all the stories she had heard about Mena. Of course, Mena wasn't diagnosed as being Bipolar, but she had all the signs of it.

Ivy's Memories

Ivy was Mena's baby sister who she was very fond of. Her name was special. In ancient Greece, newlyweds wore ivy wreaths to show their loyalty and devotion to one another. Ivy was the first to get married out of all Mena's siblings. Ivy had a quiet demeanor, and yet in all, she was the most outspoken. Ivy's name was fitting. It represents not easily letting go of something it attaches itself to. She was like a climbing evergreen plant. She would wrap herself around anyone who graciously showed love towards her.

Mena loved her babysitter because she seemed warm and innocent. Mena showed a slight jealousy over Ivy because she seemed to be Daddy's girl. Ivy would follow him around the house whenever she got a chance, too. She would cuddle up with him whenever he took a nap. When he watched football, she would be right by his side, cheering on the Colts Team. Paton was one of their favorite players. There was a picture of Ivy and her dad hanging on the wall showing them at a Dallas football game. That was one of Lisa's favorite pictures of both of them. When Ivy was ten years old, Mena was sixteen years old. They didn't play together very much because Mena was well into her friends. They were never in the same school together. Ivy and her middle sister, April, were the best of friends. They did everything together, and Chris, of course, was only six years old and off into his world with his best friend, Michael, who played with dinosaurs and wrestling men in Chris's bedroom all the time.

Somehow, Ivy still seemed to draw Mena's affection towards her. They very seldom argued. When Mena told Ivy to do something, she normally did. Ivy could be very sneaky with some things and get away with it. Mena thought Ivy was a very funny child because she was always falling, tripping over something, or falling into something. One time, she fell into a huge bucket, and all you could see were her dangling legs hanging out, crying out for Daddy. Mena thought that was hilarious. She didn't even help her out. Lisa thought it was pretty funny, too, but her motherly instinct pulled her out.

Ivy didn't remember Mena going to the hospital that often until Mena was well out of the house and married. Mena didn't mind taking care of Ivy when she was little because Ivy was full of laughter and hugs. Ivy even tried to take care of Mena when she would see Mena crying for some unknown reason. However, Mena would cry so much about so many things that Ivy would sometimes ignore her. It could be an argument with her parents or disappointment from her boyfriend, but it didn't matter. Ivy would give her big sister a gentle smile and just walk away. Ivy grew up wanting to be a good mother. Lisa knew that she would be a great wife and mother someday. Ivy ended up being an extraordinary wife and mother. Ivy loved her children very much, and she was so attached to them that whenever she left for work early, she would never leave them with the babysitters, but she would go and pick them up right away. She read them stories, played games with them, and took them out on outings whenever an opportunity arose. Lisa felt that she was a perfect example of what a mother should be, as well as caring for others. What is so ironic about the matter is that Ivy grew up working in the medical field, taking care of patients in need.

Ivy didn't have much to say about Mena and her ways. She just thought that Mena was living a normal life. Ivy didn't have Sickle Cell or Sickle Cell trait. Ivy's embryo had managed not to inherit that awful trait. Now that Ivy was older, she had realized why Mena was going through so many highs and lows like a roller coaster. Ivy had to encounter patients at the hospital who had Sickle Cell. She would sometimes have to put catheters or special ports in for plasmapheresis (a therapeutic intervention that involves extracorporeal removal, temporarily replacing a vital organ or removal of exogenous poisons), return, or exchange of blood plasma or components.

When Mena was admitted to the hospital, Ivy would drop in and visit her big sister. Not as often as she should, because Mena visited the hospital so often that Ivy had become desensitized to the visits. She was so busy at work that she often felt that Mena would be okay if she didn't visit every time she was admitted. There were times when the doctors or nurses would call Ivy personally to calm Mena down when they felt threatened or didn't know what to do with her. Sometimes it seemed so bad to the nurses that they would have what seemed like a posse of nurses in the room at one time to try to calm Mena down and administer her medication, which wasn't in the form she preferred. She didn't want a pill form but wanted them to be administered in the IV.

Ivy would say to Mena, "If you continue to be mean to the nurses, they will take their time to take care of you. You have got to stop acting this way. They can't give you the best of care if they feel threatened in some way or if you are disrespecting them. You wish this pain on all their families. You've got to calm yourself down and stop firing the doctors and nurses."

Ivy would speak to her sister as gently as she could. Ivy was trying to be as sympathetic as she could with Mena, but at times it was extremely hard to de-escalate Mena's temper. Ivy could be very oversensitive and touchy when Mena would demean her and try to talk down to her. Sometimes it just came to a point and time to let go and let Mena have to pay for the consequences of her actions. In the meantime, Ivy just felt sorry for her because Mena would just choke her words out. Ivy loved her sister so much, but sometimes there was just no way of reaching her. She would check in on her later as she had done before.

April's Memories

April was Mena's middle sister. As a newborn baby, she smelled like flowers when she arrived home from the hospital. Mena didn't like the way April looked from the moment she arrived. A streak of jealousy was already planted in Mena's heart. She had been an only child for almost four years, and here was this baby trying to take her place. Mena didn't like the color of April's almond skin or the soft, flowing hair that lay upon the top of her new baby's head. All the attention was now focused on this new baby. Mena wanted them to take her back. She now had to share a room with someone. She was no longer the only child. How dare this baby spoil it all? The older the baby got, the angrier Mena seemed to get. April never seemed to want to do anything Mena would tell her to do. They never seemed to get along. In Greek, April means the Goddess of Love. Mena felt that there was no love found anywhere in her sister. Mena was wrong; all April wanted was love from her oldest sister. She constantly tried to show affection towards Mena, but for some reason, Mena just felt that April was annoying. There were times when they did get along, and these were some of the happiest days for April. She wanted to be so much like her sister. April felt that Mena was a walking encyclopedia. She could go to Mena and gather all the information she needed if she had a question when her mom was busy walking around the house. As they got older, when Mena was seventeen and April was thirteen, they strayed even further apart, so April and Ivy continued to be the best of friends. It was as if she had become the big sister to Ivy.

Mena had other interests, as teenage girls often do, especially a boy whom she seemed to love very much. April remembers only her sister being sick or in pain from Sickle Cell a few times. There were times when she knew that Mena would go to the hospital for pain, but she would always come back and recover. Mena would experience many sudden changes in her attitude. It could be a sudden reaction to something or an extreme change in a short time. Mena's emotions could change rapidly, like a roller coaster. April just didn't have time to be bothered with Mena's mood swings. April didn't think much about what was happening to Mena at the time because she was too busy helping Mena care for and love her son, Mario, whom she loved very much.

Years later, it wasn't the physical pain that affected Mena, but the mental pain from what Mario brought into her life. Mario loved his mother deeply, but it was hard for both of them to express their love for one another, especially as Mario grew older. They used silence to keep their fragile bond intact—but there was nothing beautiful about it. However, that was the way they kept their mother-and-son relationship under control.

April knew that Mena went through cramps, swelling of her feet, and excruciating pain. She knew that this would send her in and out of the hospital. She knew that Mena could be in the hospital for weeks, so to see her like that was heartbreaking. They didn't live remarkably close to one another in their adulthood. She would often think of her cousin Autumn, who had Sickle Cell as well, and she never quite understood why she couldn't go swimming. The fact remains that it was heartbreaking as well, because that was something April loved doing: swimming at the beach. When April would peer above the water, she would watch the sadness on Mena's and Autumn's faces because she knew that they wanted to be a part of the enjoyment as well. She felt as though this was upsetting for them. They couldn't do the normal things that people did during the summer. April felt that some people didn't understand the impact Sickle Cell had on people's lives, including herself, until now, as an adult. April felt that some people consider certain things, such as this, to be common, while others consider it deadly. Swimming could make them go into a crisis. She knew that when she was younger, she didn't have a lot of emotions about what was going on with Mena, but now she knows Sickle Cell can be deadly. She knew that she was oblivious to what was going on in Mena's and Autumn's lives.

April thought about when she went to the prom with her cousin, Mark. He held up to his name, which means polite and kind. He would always speak politely and never ignore her. He always made time for her, unlike her sister Mena, who often ignored her. April would often go to his house to play. She never saw him go into a crisis. All she knew was that he had Sickle Cell too, and a few years later, he died. So, when she looked back at her prom pictures and saw them together, it made her sad, and it was heartbreaking to know that he was no longer with them. April knew that she had the trait and that it didn't affect her as much as Mena, Autumn, and Mark, but it did cause her anemia. All she knew was that she would get cold easily, and she felt like she got sick often from it, but not to the point where she needed to go to the hospital. Some doctors would disagree with that statement; they feel that those with the trait go on to live normal lives.

April remembered Mena's adult years. She remembered times when Mena wasn't strong enough and was unable to take care of her daughter, Bree, when she was five years old. She and her husband took care of her for 8 months. She was able to help her out and allow Mena to have some kind of reprieve from the stress of being in the hospital and not being able to be home with her children. Boxer, Mena's youngest son, even had to spend some time staying with his Uncle and Aunt for a time. Mario and Amelia, Mena's oldest son and daughter, stayed with their grandmother, Mum Mum. It made April feel like she knew that it helped Mena to be at ease to know that her children were in good hands.

At the same time, she also knew that Mena felt she was a horrible mom, but April knew that wasn't true. She knew that Mena couldn't help it when she was sick. It just limited her ability to be an effective parent during her absence. She knew that Mena had done what she felt was best for her children at the time. She had done what was in the best interest of her children. When Mena was admitted to the hospital in Baltimore, she would try to go and visit Mena with Bree as often as she could, just so that Mena didn't have to be alone.

Mena felt differently; she felt that being alone wasn't all that bad. It gave her time for meditation and time to cry over all that was going on in her life, without anyone noticing or asking questions like, 'How can I help you?' What can I do to make it better?

Mena would think to herself, *"Absolutely nothing unless you can absorb this pain or take it away from me."*

Mena once told April that the hospitals across the bridge were the best and had the best hospital food that she had ever tasted. It made Mena happy. Mena would never get the food that was on the hospital menu. She would order food from the Junior Board or the lunchroom. They would cater to her wishes. There were always cakes, a variety of fruits, plenty of fruit drinks, and well-made sandwiches, which Mena ordered the cooks to create. Nothing was simple when Mena arrived at the hospital. If she was going to be in pain and feeling miserable, let her last meal make her feel better. April felt that if Mena were to die, at least she would have a little bit of happiness before Sickle Cell ended her life or the complications it caused her body. April had become desensitized to that part of death itself. She prefers not to think about Mena's blood count dropping and parts of her body malfunctioning. She was oblivious to what was going on around her anyway.

I'm happy to say that now all of Mena's children are residing with her. The older kids, Mario and Amelia, are old enough to take care of Bree and Boxer when Mena has to stay at the hospital for a lengthy period. They are helping to take care of themselves because they are now fourteen and fifteen years old. April felt that with all that Mena had gone through, her kids were strong and independent, and Mena had done her best to be a good parent. April felt that she really couldn't remember stories worth mentioning about Mena and her Sickle Cell Crisis when she was younger. She just couldn't remember.

She didn't even know that Mena had Sickle Cell or experienced the pain of it until Mena was older. All she can remember now are the stories that Mena would put out on Facebook. On her Facebook page, Mena was crying as she tried to encourage people to check their genes.

Mena was saying, "Before you get together with the opposite sex, check your genes."

April remembered the way she felt. She was so proud of her sister. She was proud that Mena was very vulnerable about opening up. It was through her weaknesses that Mena was able to spread awareness. April felt that Mena was, unfortunately, the stepping stone for people to understand more about the disease of Sickle Cell.

April didn't want another baby in this world to have to grow up and or not grow up, and experience the pain that she is going through. April felt that her advice was that people should look it up. They should want to have more knowledge about it, including herself. She remembered a student who wanted to attend college with her, but he knew he would have to drop out of school and return home because his mom wouldn't want him to be far away from her. He couldn't even go to the college of his choice. He had to stay close to home so that he could be taken care of during times of crisis. The mom made a comment based on what he had at a board meeting, but neglected to say what it was; however, April knew what he had based on what the mom had mentioned. The mom wanted it to be confidential. It wasn't something she stated that the staff would be able to know, except for the nurse. Not even the student wanted anyone to know. She knew of two students who felt that way. April knew that this was something that shouldn't be hidden. People should become aware of it. If they were to voice their concerns, there would be more help given to them and their families.

April knew that those who have a voice should say it out loud: "I am a Sickle Cell Warrior." Their voices need to be heard instead of them saying "Nobody's Listening to Me If Only They Could C Me." April once again felt that she needed to research and become more familiar with information on Sickle Cell Disease. It's better late than never. April feels, just like Mena, that those in the medical field should educate themselves on this topic because they should give their patients the proper care that they deserve. This is a common frustration expressed by patients with Sickle Cell, especially since Sickle Cell isn't as pervasive as cancer or COVID-19. So, they say take this or take that as if it were a touch of the flu. Then they send them on their merry way when they need to be treated in the hospital longer.

April thought the hospital visits were quite long, but they would chat, talk, and laugh, something they hardly ever did when they were growing up together. It made a world of difference in April's life to know that they had truly become sisters. They had finally bonded together. They shared their experiences about their lives. They talked about their pains and heartbreaks. They had explained their feelings about their childhood and their adult life. They had found sisterhood at last. They had become friends.

Chapter 5

The Dark Room (Moon Flower)

Moon Flower: These special plants only bloom at night, when the moon is out. During the day, moonflowers are no larger than an inch or two wide, but when the sun sets, they open up to an astounding six or seven inch long bloom. Because of their aloof bloom and sweet smell, moonflowers are extremely romantic. https://www.1800flowers. com In flower language, they often represent dreams, intuition, and the mysteries of the night. https://www.picturethisai.com

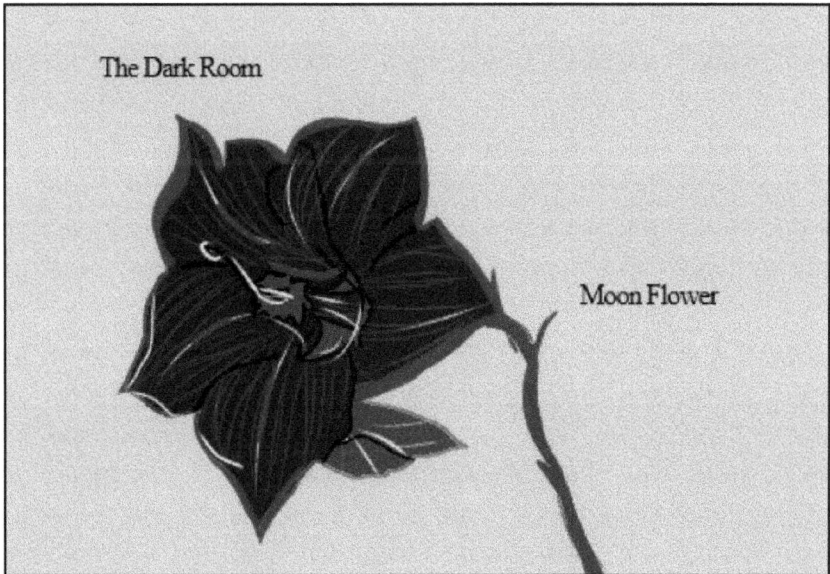

The Dark Room

Moon Flower

Something To Explore

Boxer entered the dark, musty room. The room had a mildewy and moldy aroma. It smelled like there was no ventilation and a buildup of dust and grime. Boys tend to like that smell. It was a part of their nature. There was nothing sweet-smelling about the Dark Room where Boxer's mom lay most of the time. It smelled nothing like the fragrance of the bloomed Moonflowers that his mother had arranged along the sidewalk, leading to the front door of the house. The flowers were truly a mystery to Boxer, something to explore. The Moon flowers lay flopped over during the day and opened up seven inches tall when the moon appeared. Once he entered the house, he went straight to his mother's room. He was always excited to see his mother. His mother would play games with him when she had the time and was feeling well. He was hoping that maybe this would be the time. His mom's room seemed so adventurous. He felt as though the dark room was a place for him to go scavenger hunting. Boxer thought he would discover something old and antique in the room, hoping it would have something of value.

He said to himself, "*I am going to be the richest boy in the world.*" He just knew that if he became the richest boy in the world, he would start a foundation that would find a cure for whatever it was that was plaguing his mother daily, weekly, and sometimes monthly.

Scavenger Hunt

Boxer turned his attention back to his mother's darkroom. Looking around with his magnifying glass, he was sure there was a hidden treasure that had been placed somewhere. Boxer looked for cracks in the flooring. He looked under a pile of laundry that was on the floor. Mena hadn't had the strength to take care of any housework. He looked underneath the old antique dresser that was in the room with his flashlight. He was sure he would find something there. Only to find cobwebs. He thought to himself, "*Maybe it's camouflaged. It's possible it is blending in with part of the room. Could it be hidden inside something? Like her jewelry box, or behind the dark curtains.*" He had totally forgotten how excited he was about coming to see his mother to play a game with her. He had forgotten about why his mother was in the room in the first place, lying in the darkness, groaning and moaning with excruciating pain. Mena was just like a moonflower most of the time. She would come out of her room when the sun was beginning to set and go back into her dark room by midday.

I Spy

Boxer shouted out, "Mommy, why don't we play I spy? I want to hunt for a hidden treasure!"

Mena replied, "Oh, I would love to, Boxer, but I am in too much pain to play. I need rest and some sleep. I promise we will play another day."

Boxer stood there in disappointment and said, "Okay, Mommy." Mena yelled in horrifying pain. Boxer quickly responded with a caring heart, "Are you okay, Mommy?"

Mena answered him with all the words she could muster up and said, "We can play later, okay, now you go run and play."

Boxer left the room, wondering if his mommy would get better soon so that he could play I Spy and find that ancient artifact in the Dark Room. He knew that one day he would be a great archaeologist. In his mind, he knew that an archaeologist uncovered the unknown, and he was determined to find something. That would be his career in life. His thoughts reverted to his mom, filled with so much love for her, and he hoped that soon she would step out of that dark room into the light. He would be waiting for that play date of "I Spy." Boxer's insides were burning with sadness and excitement. He was excited that he got to see his mother and that she had promised him that they would play "I Spy" another day. At the same time, he was sad that he was unable to find that hidden treasure to make things all the better for his mom.

Mena stayed in the dark often because she seemed to be losing her vision. In the light, she saw spots in front of her eyes. Thoughts of blindness were constantly looming in her brain. It was like seeing an abstract picture with black circles all the time, so she preferred to visit the dark room often, along with the pain that kept her there.

Chapter 6

I Want to Go Home
(Monarch Butterfly)

Insects such as the monarch butterfly regularly migrate thousands of miles to and from their breeding grounds, and many other species navigate effectively over shorter distances. Memory plays a significant role for those who make multiple round trips over a lifetime. That's obviously impossible in short-lived species. That means long-distance navigation must involve an innate ability to use environmental cues. Monarch butterflies migrate from North America to specific trees in Mexico (up to 3,000km) every autumn. https://discoverwildlife.com

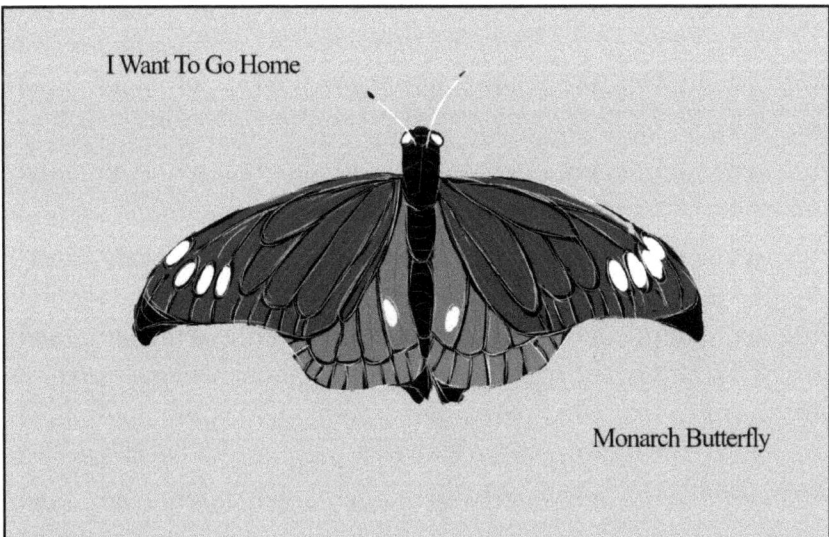

I Want To Go Home

Monarch Butterfly

Amelia Losing Her Best Friend

Amelia found it exceedingly difficult to live with her mother during her teenage years. Her mom was happy one moment and angry the next. When she was healthier, Mena was the best mom in the world. She was interested in everything that the kids were interested in. Her Sickle Cell was much milder then. Now, she was even more tired, so she took many naps, and she was very restless. Mena's trips to the hospital were more frequent. Growing up was hard for Amelia and Mario. Amelia felt that once her mother had two more siblings, Bree and Boxer, there was too much on her body that was filled with Sickle Cells, and it took a turn for the worse.

Amelia would say, "Mom, what are we going to do today? Let's go to the mall and shop until we drop."

Mena would say, "No, not today; I'm feeling extra tired."

Amelia began to notice that her mom was always tired. The house was clean, but it always seemed as if Mena was exhausted from something more than cleaning the house.

Amelia began to wonder and said, "Mom, what's wrong with you? All you want to do is sit on the couch like a couch potato and watch the Soap Operas all day long. You used to be my best friend. We used to go out all the time and have a wonderful time. You know I don't have any friends here. I am so bored. I want to go home."

Mena would reply, "You are home. Maybe you should try and go make some friends and stop acting weird."

Amelia acted somewhat strange to the kids at her school. Her mother didn't understand why Amelia didn't want to make new friends, because she knew they wouldn't live there for long. They would move, and she would have her heart broken all over again by moving away from the friends she had made. They would move on to another adventure, somewhere else. They would never see their close friends ever again, so why try? Anyway, being the new girl wasn't exciting because most of the kids had established their friends. Amelia felt as if she would be the tag-along. Amelia yelled, "I want to go and live with my Mum Mum."

Moving Away

Two months later, the family moved to Arizona. It was extremely hot there. Amelia wondered if the weather was causing her mom's sickness. *Was the weather making her sick and tired all the time?* She watched her mom drink more and more water as if the water were seeping through all the layers of her skin. It was as if no matter how much she drank, her body just couldn't contain it. Mena's Sickle Cell attacks were getting worse. It was as if her Sickle Cells were multiplying more and more. Not only was Mena sleeping a lot, but she was going to the hospital more often. All Amelia could picture in her head now was her mother being connected to an IV, getting fluid pushed through her body, and it was a lot of moaning and groaning with pain attached to it. It was time to move back to the Carolinas because Mena's body seemed to be getting extremely worse.

They had lived in a lot of places: Arizona, Kentucky, Colorado, Carolina, Maryland, Virginia, Texas, and twice in Georgia. There was one place Amelia loved. She called it her place of Paradise, the lake house. She could hear Empire was streaming on the TV, but nothing could take the place of hearing the sounds of the beautiful lake. However, the lake house would become another memory loss. Something that Amelia would keep stored up in her brain. They would also leave the lake house. The memories of it would become a part of her past. Amelia's thoughts began to become overly dramatic, fueled by her imagination.

When they had moved to the next house, it seemed as if a ghost had lived there in Amelia's mind. No kids were playing in the neighborhood. The house was always dark, and her mom spent most of her time in the Dark Room, as Boxer called it. The master bedroom, to Amelia, felt like it was moist, dreary, and sickly, with barely any windows. There were only two tiny ones where the light hardly ventures in at all. Her parents had a king bed. Amelia couldn't remember much else about the room because it was too dark. It was a garage that someone had turned into a bedroom. Amelia couldn't even remember where the light switches were because the light bothered her mother and prevented her from getting a good night's sleep. All that room did was just take her mother's breath away. It was as if the room had spread to the house itself. The house was dark and airy. There was no Wi-Fi, no cable.

Sometimes, Amelia and Mario would walk to Barnes & Noble just so they could get Wi-Fi. In Amelia's mind, she would say, "Mario and I have played Sky Room over a million times. It's kind of boring to use this as a source of entertainment."

They would read comic books, history books, and scary books — simply different books at Barnes & Noble. They were tired of reading the same books over and over again at home. Their mom wasn't there to help them exchange them.

Amelia thought to herself, *"I have read these books at the house over six times, and I don't even like reading, so that says a lot."*

The room had a back door that led to the backyard, where no one wanted to play. It was full of poop from the dog, and briars were all over the yard. It just wasn't the right room for her mom. Amelia began to think about the bad memories in her life, like when the laundry was piling up and there was no food in the house because her mom was in the hospital for days, weeks, or even a month at a time.

Breaking Down Of The Family

Amelia began noticing that a series of events were just happening, and things just started to get dramatic and messy, and with that, stress came along, causing her mom to go into a Sickle Cell Crisis. Mario stayed in his room. Bree and Boxer accepted all the strength and time Mena could give. Amelia and her mother no longer shared many things, so Amelia began to withdraw within herself. Amelia had begun feeling depressed, just like her mother.

Mena was not only going through a Sickle Cell Crisis, but she was also going through the breakdown of her family. Mena and her husband, Rex, never seemed to see eye to eye. They were always yelling and screaming at one another. All Mena wanted was love and support, especially when she had to go to the hospital. Having her children's affection was just not enough.

Amelia thought to herself, *"Mommy's always gone to the hospital. I can't check in on her like I want to. I'm not old enough to drive."*

Amelia was so worried about when her mother would be coming back. Amelia spoke out loud, "I wish Bree and Boxer would quit asking me questions because I don't know the answers." The whole house reminded her of the song: "Ain't no sunshine when she's gone 'cause she's always gone too long, anytime she goes away."

Amelia thought to herself, *"Mommy always did the laundry and grocery shopping."*

They weren't able to go to the food pantry. Mena would take them, and they would get lots of food there that would fill the house. Mario and Amelia first started drinking a lot of coffee because there wasn't enough food in the house to go around. It helped to fill their stomachs. They loved Bree and Boxer, so they would let them eat to ensure their growing bodies had enough nourishment to last throughout the day. They would just scrap things together, eat a lot of noodles, or eat lots of things together, or eat numerous peanut butter and jelly sandwiches. Amelia hates peanut butter and jelly, as well as noodles, to this day. It wasn't that their parents didn't have the money; it was just that Mena took care of all the household tasks and finances. Buying groceries was one of them. Amelia felt sad about not being able or old enough to take care of her little brother and sister the way she wanted to. Amelia didn't understand many things that were happening at the house. Things were just getting out of control. Mena would try to take care of the family from the hospital, issuing orders over the phone, but Amelia felt that it just wasn't working at all. It only caused Mena more stress, and them as well. The kids were doing the best they could without their mother being there, but their best wasn't good enough.

Amelia would say, "My sensitive spot has been touched." Amelia meant that her heart was aching, and she wasn't an emotional person. She began to cry silently.

Mena would say to Amelia, "Are the kids okay? Are they eating well?"

The kids kept secrets from their mom because they didn't want her to know the true story and what was really going on. They knew that if she did, she would come home immediately that very night in pain. So, they kept their mouths shut. Amelia remembered a morning when they were hungry and she couldn't find Rex. She looked out the window of the house, and there was Rex. He was sitting in his car, eating a bowl of cereal, knowing that they hadn't been fed and that there was no food in the house.

Amelia thought out loud, "I suppose Rex is doing what he can do best, and at the same time, he said, 'I need to work to provide for you guys.' There were times when he would hang out with his friends, and they wouldn't see him until the next day. He said, 'It was to relieve his stress.'

Rex gambled a lot. We would hear mommy and Rex arguing because he would gamble his paycheck at the Casino or play the lottery. Later, he would come home and brag about the things that he had brought. He would say, 'Kids, come and look at what I bought! Do you like my new watch? Let me show you how it works. Hey kids, I bought you a 70-inch TV.' The following week, the TV would be gone from where he had lost money and had to pay someone back, or lost it to his gambling habits.

Rex was like a kid at heart. He loved playing with gadgets. He loved anything that dealt with technology. I remembered him going inside my computer and fixing the memory in it. He could build a whole computer if he needed to. He was very smart in that sense, but taking care of the family was something that just wasn't quite built into him. We all had a lot of fun with him from time to time.

Bree and Boxer loved him most. Even Mario and Amelia sometimes thought he was cool, but they were old enough to know that he wasn't the best father when it came to meeting the family's essential needs.

Ameila knew that Rex wasn't the best husband in the world either. Amelia would overhear her mother talking to her parents, Lisa and Bruce, asking them for money just to put food on the table. Her mom would be crying and stressing out from the pain that Rex was causing her. Amelia knew that stress caused her mother to go into crisis, so she would help her mom in any way she could.

Some weeks, Mena would say, "Hand over your paycheck so that I can pay the bills and buy some groceries."

Rex would say, "I don't have it. I tried to make more money with it. Ask your parents to help us out. You don't have any problems when

I do win. I'm the one working in this family, so I should be able to do what I want with my money."

Mena would reply, "I thought you once said, what's yours is mine. Do you remember that? You left it up to me to make a budget for this family. I can't budget what I don't have." Then the back-and-forth yelling would begin.

Amelia Has Enough

Amelia didn't know how to do laundry very well, and when her eyes gazed upon all the dirty laundry piling up, she felt every muscle in her body ache. She wasn't the best cook, either; however, she did know how to make grilled cheese sandwiches and spaghetti when her mother was away at the hospital and when Rex was who knows where. She felt a thirteen-year-old should not have to handle all this. Amelia had had enough.

When Amelia finally couldn't take it any longer, Amelia picked up the phone and called: "Hi, Mum Mum, I miss you. I want to come back home."

Lisa was on pins and needles to hear the reason why. She had missed Amelia so much. It was like having a second chance at raising Mena all over again. Amelia was a spitting image of her mother from the day she was born. Amelia looked so much like Mena when she was a baby. Lisa could hardly tell their pictures apart. Amelia was a joy to have, and she was always by her side, tagging along. Amelia helped alleviate some of the loneliness Lisa felt when her husband was at work all day and her son, Chris, was at his best friend Michael's house. She didn't have that sense of loneliness when Amelia was around. Lisa thought about Amelia as being a monarch butterfly. Monarchs can represent transformation and rebirth to some people. They might view a monarch's sighting as a sign of an upcoming change or a new direction in their life.

Lisa asked herself, *"Is my life and Amelia's life about to change and go into a new direction?"* Lisa asked, "What's wrong?"

Amelia answered Mum Mum and said, "Mommy is always sleeping or in the hospital, and all I feel like I am nothing but a babysitter. I'm tired of moving all over the place. Every time I make a friend, we move, and our friendship ends. I have no friends here. Mum Mum, there's no place like home. Please come and get me."

Meds taking a toll on Mena

"Mum Mum, at dinner last night, my mom fell asleep, and her head fell smack into the mashed potatoes. She was unable to function. Her entire body just gave way. When she woke up, she had mashed potatoes on her nose. The doctors are giving my mom such large doses of medicine, and I don't feel like they should be doing that to a person. Mommy is a completely different person when she is on her meds. She just walks around the house, vigorously cleaning and wandering. We can't control the things that she does. It's as if she doesn't even acknowledge us or know who we are. In some ways, I know that Mom needs it, but maybe not in such high doses. The medicine is taking a toll on her. I was thinking she might need it, but there has to be a natural remedy for it. That's what I have read in some books at Barnes & Noble. I like reading about history and medical things. Someday I want to be a Naturopathic doctor. I want to help my mom. My grades are failing because we never stay at one school long enough. I was in a special nursing program at the last school I attended, but it is not offered at the school I am attending now. It's affecting Mario and me, but Bree and Boxer are still too young to notice that this is not normal, the way Mom is behaving, and that it is affecting them. I've tried to help her as much as I can, as a matter of fact, we all have, but Mum Mum, I'm just a teenager," Amelia began to cry, "I don't want to be here anymore."

Chapter 7

Moving (Wild Sunflower)

The domestic sunflower, however, often possesses only a single large inflorescence (flower head) atop an unbranched stem. It is commonly grown as a crop for its edible oily seeds. They can be used as an ornament in domestic gardens. Distribution and habitat: The precise native range is difficult to determine. Regardless of its original range, it can now be found in almost every part of the world that is not tropical, desert, or tundra- https://en.wikipedia.org

Lisa was lying in bed after a sleepless night of spending too much time on her iPhone looking at and listening to the thoughts and videos that were on Facebook. It is amazing how you can get caught up in someone's problems and happiness all at once. She had finally fallen off to sleep, and her husband awakened her after feeding Sock the cat. Bruce walked over and rubbed her back ever so gently. Bruce knew a morning rub always started Lisa's day in the best way possible.

It reminded her of Mena when she would say, "Don't stop, Daddy, don't stop."

At the age of 65, Lisa knew that it was enjoyable for him as well because she knew that her brown skin was still as smooth as a baby's skin. No lumps, bumps, or wrinkles. She knew he loved her brown skin. Lisa would say, "Good morning, honey. That feels so good. Can you rub a little longer this morning?"

Bruce replied, "Sure, baby, I can do that."

The TV had been left on all night, and the news was on. She could hear a man's gentle voice talking about Wild Sunflowers.

Lisa turned over and sat up and said, "Honey, I have got to rewind that and hear the poetry about the Wildflowers again. It reminds me so much of Mena. It was one of the most beautiful poems I have ever heard in a long time."

Bee used to read poems to Lisa all the time. She loved to hear Bee's gentle voice as she lay across Bee's bed in comfort. It soothed her soul with peace. I loved Bee's name. The name Bee means A person of integrity. It symbolizes hard work and diligence, much like a Bee working for its queen. They were just teenagers then, and now Bee is a famous poet. Bruce got up and went into the bathroom, following his usual routine. Lisa grabbed the black control with eagerness to hear the poem again. She replayed the poem at least eight times to write down every line. Mena was on her mind with every line she heard.

Wild Sunflowers

Lisa was listening to Charles Paparella on WBOC, quoting a poem. It was just beautiful. One of the things he said was that we have an abundance of yellow around the Delmarva. He was speaking of the Wild Flower. He spoke of the Wild Sunflowers that are everywhere. He mentioned how the Sunflowers that grow along the cornfields, along the ditch banks, take over the whole field. If you've seen pictures of HbSC images, they look pretty. However, they take over a whole person's body as they had done to Mena's body. He mentioned how they celebrate the sun. "I fear that there is no celebration for Mena, because all the sun does at times is dehydrate Mena's body, which causes her to go into a crisis." In the poem, it suggests that not all flowers show their devotion, such as the Moon Flower, to the central power of the source, which is the sun. Sad to say, Mena felt like she was the moonflower. The moon only loves the moon flower. The moon was like her family - the only ones who truly loved her. This was definitely such an obviousness of sadness. This was not true at all; there were others who loved Mena. Depression had put her in that zone. One verse said, "The moon didn't care for those who loved the sun; it gives them no comfort." Lisa compared that line to the doctors, who gave Mena no comfort in seeing her in the light of day. During the nighttime, the Sunflowers are scared, so they cover their eyes, and they are happy when the sun returns. Mena, in her own world of darkness, feels comfort where she is able to open her eyes to doctors and share her knowledge of Sickle Cell, so she waits until the next morning in daylight. The SunFlowers' fear is being replaced with joy and smiles as the sun returns. For Mena, her fear begins as the sun rises, and her smile is just a smile turned upside down. The night has come to an end, and she must bring attention. A change "has got to come" with educating doctors about different forms of Sickle Cell and the treatment for each form, just as the Sunflowers bring their attention to changes in hue.

A Beautiful Place

Mena's family was like a Sunflower. They never knew where they would be living from year to year. She could live almost anywhere except in extremely hot climates. She had to keep her body dehydrated. She was so excited about moving down south or to a place like Hawaii, but the elevated temperature ranges of 90 degrees to 100 degrees were just too much for her body. Mena and her family had moved at least ten times by now. She found that either the neighborhood of people or the environmental climate did not work for her. Most of her housing was apartment living. Mena and Rex had moved into a house in Augusta, Georgia—a beautiful place where there was a pond in her backyard.

Mena would come out and talk to all the animals and birds that lived there. "Good morning, my Osprey friend. It is about time you came and visited me this morning. We can have our breakfast together. I am having tea and a muffin this morning. What are you having? I suppose you're having fish and a few beetle bugs. That sounds great for you, but not for me, thank you. Maybe some other time. I am sure your diet contributes to a long life, and you consistently demonstrate loyalty and wisdom. You never miss a meal, and you always know where your habitat is. I wish I could say the same. With this Sickle Cell residing within me, I don't know where I am going to live from month to month or year to year. I hope this will be the place I will live in for the rest of my life. This feels like home. I dream of the meaning of your name, my Osprey friends. Your name means grace, devotion, faithfulness, open-mindedness, aspiration, longevity, immortality, and transformation. Even though I know a lot of the meanings of your name are symbolic, I want all those qualities. When I think about it, in a way, we are so much alike, and then again, not so much alike. Longevity and immortality are not in the cards for me. My heart strives for eternity; however, this Sickle Cell Disease gives me a check every morning, saying I am going to take you out. While you stand there on one leg, alarming your children of the danger that is ahead of them, I, too, someday will have to alert my children that it is time to move on."

The Alarming Day

That alarming day did come; it was time to move on. The elevation of the area was too much for Mena's body to withstand. She often spent her time in and out of the hospital.

Her body could not take it any longer, and she had to break the news to the children. Bree and Boxer had just come from playing down by the dock, where they would often visit their turtle friend, Ninja. Mena needed to just breathe before she had to break the awful news to them. Bree and Boxer knew by the expression on their mother's face that something was wrong.

Bree said, "Mommy, what's wrong?"

Mena replied, "We have to move again. The elevation of the mountains is too high for my body."

Boxer screamed at his mother, "But Mommy, I don't want to go. I like it here. This is the best place we have ever lived. We can't leave Ninja, our turtle; he's our friend. Who's going to feed him and take care of him?"

Bree cried, "Please, let's not go. We love him, Mommy. What about the new friends we have made? They are going to miss us, and we are going to miss them, too."

Boxer ran off crying to his room and slammed the door. Mena's heart was filled with disappointment that her body had inherited Sickle Cell. It was always taking control of her coming and going.

Mena looked into Bree's sad eyes and said, "Bree, you must love me more than a turtle. He will survive in the water with plenty of bugs to eat."

Bree was getting older now, and she acknowledged that her mother was right. Bree wishes she could stop how the Sickle Cell disease invaded her mother's body. Bree knew that her mother was doing the best she could. For some reason, Bree thought that her mother had it under control because they were all so happy. There was another battle Mena knew she had to fight. It was telling her oldest kids. Sometimes they fought with yelling, and then sometimes they fought with silence, especially Mario. Mena's son's name means man of war. It is of Italian origin. It also means antihero, which focuses on personal motives first and foremost, with everything else secondary. Amelia's name means "industrious" or "hardworking." Amelia was the one who kept her silence most of the time. That name perfectly suited her. She approached life with the desire to do her best. No one would get in her way of doing that. Mena had just left a hostile environment a year ago, where she used to live. She thought she had a good friend there. It was just the opposite. This place she thought was simply perfect.

Chapter 8

Sickle Cell Trait or Sickle Cell Disease "Diagnosis" (Marsh Marigold or Celandine)

Marsh Marigold can be confused with invasive Lesser Celandine. Marsh Marigolds spread easily. Lesser Celandine are shiny, dark green leaves. Their leaves are heart-to-kidney-shaped. Marsh Marigolds are also dark green, but much larger. They both spread quickly and easily.

They both occur in moist soil and are low-growing with bright yellow flowers. "Lower Hudson Prison."

The difference between a flower and a weed is a matter of your perception. People perceive them in a certain way because some plants grow in places where they don't want them to, such as your beautiful green lawn that looks and feels like carpet under your feet. It is not what the heart desires or is looking for. The flower or weed can be plants that grow quickly or that may have an extensive root system structure that spreads above or below the ground, which can be a pain in the butt for some. https://sciencing.com by Meg Michelle updated March 24,2022

The difference between a flower and a weed is analogous to the difference between Sickle Cell Disease and Sickle Cell Trait.

The Sickle Cell Care Package

Bree came home after school and said, "Mommy, look at what I got. The school gave a care package to all those who have Sickle Cell. Look, they gave me slime, hand sanitizer, bracelets, slap hands, candy, and an information sheet about Sickle Cell."

Mena looked puzzled and said, "Bree, you don't have Sickle Cell, you have Sickle Cell Trait." You know that they are both inherited blood disorders, but they are different in the severity levels and the symptoms they have, as well as how they should be treated. We discussed this before: how a person with Sickle Cell disease inherits two sickle cell genes. One from each parent. It causes their red blood cells to become hard, and they have a crescent shape. This can lead to numerous health problems. Sickle cell Trait has one gene for normal hemoglobin and one gene for sickle hemoglobin. Usually, a person doesn't have any symptoms and lives a normal life.

Bree replied, "I know, but they think I do."

At least that's what Bree was thinking they were thinking.

"They are going to give us a care package about every 2 months. Mommy, they said, that at Christmas time, the care package is going to include blankets, candy, gloves, and hats. They know that we have to stay warm so that our cells don't jam up when we are cold. That was good on their part, don't you think, Mommy?"

Mena didn't have a chance to answer because Bree had moved on to talking about the month of June's care package.

Bree continued and said, "In June, we are going to get beach towels, bubbles, sunglasses, and probably some more toys." Bree whispered, "I didn't dare tell them that most people with Sickle Cell don't go swimming. The water is much too cold for them. Like you, mommy, your cells jam every time you go swimming. It's just too strenuous for your body and way too cold for you."

Boxer looked confused and said, "Bree, how come you got a care package, and I didn't? I have Sickle Cell Trait too."

Obviously, the school wasn't aware that Boxer was diagnosed with Sickle Cell Trait. No one had ever asked him, and Mena had never told the administration or the nurse, because it wouldn't have affected his education in school. Braylah was more outspoken about things in her life, and she had mentioned it to her teacher. So, without investigating Bree's diagnosis, they started giving her packages as well.

Bree gave Boxer a teenager's look of frustration, "I don't know; you'll have to ask your teacher."

Then she skipped off happily and excitedly. Mena was in one of those moods where she just didn't feel like discussing the importance of Bree's school, not knowing the difference between Sickle Cell disease and Sickle Cell Trait. It could have been that Bree was confused about what they did know.

Mena didn't want to spoil Bree's jolly moment as she had done several times in the past. So, she said to herself, "I will just deal with it later."

However, Boxer was not finished with wanting his question to be answered. So, he asked the question again, this time more persistently, "Mommy, why didn't I get a care package?"

Mena found herself struggling to deal with the matter that was at hand. She could feel the stress of the day interfering with the logic she so strongly wanted to impart to her son when answering his question reasonably. What was the reason? Mena could feel herself going into another crisis. She could feel the pain building up as the day continued. The only answer she could come up with was "Boxer, I will call your teacher tomorrow to see that you get one."

Boxer was satisfied with the answer he was given. He smiled and just ran off to play on the PlayStation in his room. Mena smiled at seeing the smile on her son's face. Mena was grateful it was a temporary fix. Mena felt gloomy inside because she knew that she wanted to give him more of a justified answer, but just couldn't at that moment. Mena also knew deep down that that phone call was not going to happen tomorrow. Mena's meds were about to kick in, and she most likely would sleep the whole night and all tomorrow. If Mena's meds didn't relieve her from the pain that she was encountering, she would surely have to go to the Hospital. She hated her hometown hospital. Mena felt as though they were incompetent when it came to her care. It would be another day of not being there for her children when they needed her.

Mena's Invasive Presence At The Hospital

Sometimes she could be like a Celandine Flower-invasive. The doctors and nurses seemed not to want her there at the hospital, as far as Mena was concerned. Everyone could feel her presence as a great advocate for herself and others who had Sickle Cell. The news of her presence would spread quickly and easily by word of mouth. Mena was known for directing the doctors and nurses about how to care for her. Mena would leave no stone unturned when it came to her care. Mena's presence made everyone on the floor feel uncomfortable. She had fired many of the doctors who were in her care. Their knowledge about Sickle Cell was very limited, especially when it came to HbSC (Hemoglobin Sickle Cell).

Mena was a little stressed out and thought back on this situation with Bree's school, and she was a little confused about what had just happened. If the school gave Bree information on Sickle Cell, why don't they know the difference between Sickle Cell Disease and Sickle Cell Trait? Mena said to herself, "That's a battle I will have to think about and deal with later. Bree could have been mistaken. Mena was so tired of fighting and explaining. Mena felt that the moment she discovered she had HbSC (Hemoglobin Sickle Cell) disease, she was always having to explain and fight battles, especially when it came to explaining how different individuals react differently. It depends on what type of Sickle Cell someone may have. Today, the battle was Sickle Cell VS Sickle Cell Trait. Today was not the day. Mena decided to go and lie down. For now, her Sickle Cell Crisis was having the upper hand. She was feeling like a weed, being in a position or place where she ought not to be. She was a Celandine. Maybe just maybe a Marigold. Throughout many cultures, marigolds were thought of as a link between death and despaired love. They represented grief or despair for the loss of a loved one-most notably shown in Mexican culture as the Day of the Dead celebrations. Sometimes Mena felt that way. She was ready for the time of celebration of her death, wanting this feeling of grief and despair to go away. Mena had loved hard, and death was sure to follow. But not today.

Chapter 9

Inherited Trait (Cry Wolf)

The origin of the expression "cry wolf" comes from one of the Aesop's Fables. The Boy Who Cried Wolf. In the story, a young shepherd amuses himself by calling for help, saying a wolf is threatening his flock when nothing is really happening. He cries wolf so often that when a wolf actually menaces the flock, no one comes to help. "Don't pay attention to Peter; he's only crying wolf. https://www.gingersoftware.com

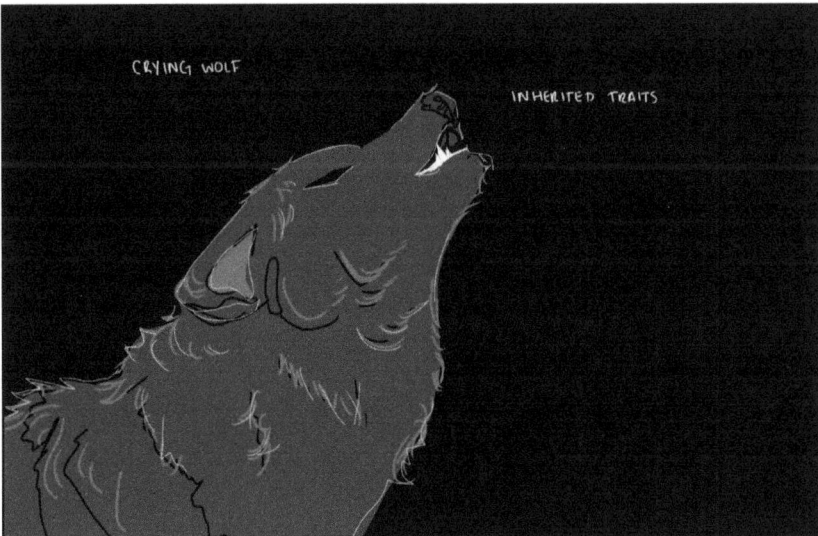

When Mario was a little boy, he remembers his mom, Mena, crying and being in pain. He would come to her aid, and his heart would skip a beat for fear that his mother was going to die. He couldn't understand why his mommy was in such pain because he didn't see anyone hitting her or any objects being thrown at her. There were times when his mother would cry when she and his daddy would be yelling at each other. He would see them pushing or shoving one another, so he knew the reason for her pain and crying. But this, this right here, was invisible to the eyes. No one was hitting, pushing, or throwing anything at his mommy. Mario would pat his mother or kiss her to help with the Boo Boo. Mommy would smile and then go back to moaning and groaning. Mario thought that he heard laughter coming from his mother from time to time, but later in life, he understood that she was crying, not laughing. Since his rubbing, hugging, and kissing his mother didn't seem to work over the years, Mario gave his mother fewer rubs, fewer hugs, and fewer kisses. His mother read him the story "The Boy Who Cried Wolf," and he related her cries to that story. The villagers had heard the boy cry wolf so many times that they no longer came to help him from the Big Bad Wolf. Finally, they stopped coming when the little boy would cry wolf. After a while, Mario's feeling of concern started to diminish. His running to his mother's cry and pain tended to be less frequent, and finally, it came to a stop. He felt overwhelmed that there was nothing he could do to help. There were times when he would come, and she would say, 'Leave me alone, I'm fine.' Mario decided to shut out her cries and make it a normal part of his life. Finally, her cries and tears became a natural part of his life. He felt absolutely nothing when she cried in pain. Eventually, that's how others felt. She would be taken to the hospital and dropped off for the doctors and nurses to comfort and take care of her. People just stopped coming. They would say to her, 'I will give you a call to check on you.' Can you let me know if you need anything? Can you let me know when you get back home? It seemed to be a natural thing to others. Everyone felt she'd be back home once she was hooked up to the IV to push her cells and given medicine. Mena had been to the hospital so many times that people weren't taking her crisis seriously anymore. Not even her family. Visits from others to see Mena became fewer and fewer.

Not a Normal Family

One day, Mena was crying out in pain, and Mario's best friend Charles said, "Should we do something?"

Charles was always concerned about what was going on in the family. His name means traveling man. It suited him well. He was like a freeman roaming about. He was a traveling man. He would always say, "I've got to start my life all over again."

He was like the words in the song, "Papa was a Rolling Stone." Wherever he laid his hat was his home. Coming and going as he pleased. However, he was overly concerned about Mena's family. Their family wasn't the normal family he had been used to.

Charles said, "I know that your mom has Sickle Cell, do something to help her out!"

Charles was Mario's best friend. He asked Mario, "Do you think that you have lived a normal life? Because, man, you're not showing any emotions, and you're acting as if you don't even care. You're not even bothering to get up to help your mom. Man, this is not normal."

Mario's answer was "My life wasn't normal because of my mom having Sickle Cell. There are so many other things. I don't know. A lot of the crazy stories about my mom are more from my mom being my mom. My cousin, Autumn, has Sickle Cell, and she doesn't have any crazy stories like my mom. I could tell you so many stories."

When Mario saw his mom going through a crisis, he would never step in to help. He was the least helpful. Out of all the members of his family, he would just disappear when his mom was in a crisis. When Mena was in pain, she would turn into an angry, irritated person. Mario wanted to avoid his mother's anger. It wasn't that he didn't care, but he mimicked anger within himself because he knew that their lives were not normal. He had missed out on so many things because his stepfather, Rex, was an emotional wreck with his PSD, and his mom seemed as if she were Bipolar. So, to avoid this strange upbringing in his life, he just decided to accept it all. It had nothing to do with the love he had for his mother when he disappeared. It had everything to do with coping.

Mario went on to tell Charles, "When she's in pain and angry. I just left her alone. She gets mad and stuff, so I will just be like, I'm going away. When she needs help or is hurting, I don't help her unless she asks me to. If she doesn't ask, I don't help. If my mom needs something while she is at the hospital, it depends on what it is; I won't be her first call. She'll call Amelia first. Because she knows if she talks to me in a crazy way, I will just say no and hang up. Then, I won't answer the phone. I don't care how angry she gets. I don't deal with that if people are going to be all mad and yelling. I'm like, nope! I will be just like hanging up. I'm not going to have people just yelling at me on the phone. Because I started acting like that, she doesn't yell at me on the phone. She doesn't ask me to do errands. She now just asks me to do things that she really wants me to do. She's not picky; what I do is what she gets. If I miss something, oh well."

Mena was known to be like a drill sergeant on the phone, yelling out directions. Do this, do that; if you don't, the yelling would begin.

Charles said, "Well, she looks like she is going to need help to get into the car. She can barely walk."

Mario replied, "Man, no matter how much she's struggling, I don't help. I can tell you that I've probably only helped my mom five times, maybe once or twice, not many times at all. I've helped her get into the car to go to the hospital, maybe once. If she don't ask, I don't do. When she is in pain, she is one angry person. She would rather do things by herself. If she were in the hospital and she asked me to do something when I was younger, I would just do it. Now that I am older, I just don't. She doesn't want you to unless she asks you to."

Charles said, "Man, that's your mom."

Mario's Helpful Ways

Mario replied, "Amelia and I do help her, especially when she is gone to the hospital. We clean and help Bree and Boxer get ready for school. There were times when Amelia and I didn't go to school. We had to stay home with the kids when Rex, our stepdad, had to go to work. We had to babysit."

"You know, Charles, I wondered if the teachers thought I was weird. They never asked me any questions. Sometimes I didn't go to school for a week. You would think that they would ask what's going on. Then, when I did go to school, I was asleep most of the time. I think one teacher asked me what was going on. She said, 'You're always tired and sleepy.' I was like, 'Leave me alone, I'm here, aren't I?' I was always tired and sleepy, that was true."

Charles said, "Why were you always tired and sleepy?"

Mario answered, "I think it started kicking in as I got older. I had a sleep problem. I'm just always sleepy; like, I could just go to sleep any time of the day. If I am somewhere comfortable, I will just go to sleep. I would take a nap to calm down when I got really angry. I would do that on purpose. You can't wake up angry from a nap. It calms you down sleeping; lowers your blood pressure."

"Lots of times, I would cook food for everyone. I would cook whatever was in there. Somebody's got to help take care of them. That's when I step in, so I'm not as cold as you may be thinking I am. My mom doesn't want help unless she tells me or asks me. So, I leave my mom alone to do whatever she's going to do. That's our family being normal.

When the kids became older, I would make them clean up after themselves. The kids try to make her go to bed when she's in pain, and I say to myself I'm not doing that. That's just too much because she is going to try to argue with you, so I'm not doing that. There were times when my mom was on some powerful meds, acting really weird, like she would be outside in the cold and wouldn't come inside. There were also times when she would fall asleep while cleaning or cooking, and the kids thought it was funny. They would say, 'Ha Ha, mommy, you're falling asleep at the counter.' They thought it was funny. It was weird, but now I'm just used to it. It doesn't really happen all the time now. That was when she was on that other medicine. That strong stuff was like she was zombified; she looked like the crackheads on the street. That's what it looked like. Like they would be huffing and rocking side to side, and their heads would be nodding back and forth. I would just lift my voice on a higher note and say, 'Just leave her alone and she'll fall asleep eventually and stay asleep.' Amelia would be like 'Mommy, Mommy.'

'I would be like Amelia, just leave her alone.'"

Charles said, "Man, I didn't know you guys were dealing with all of this."

Normal Stuff

Mario said, "You know, man, the only time I would say something or help out half the time is when she would fall asleep in the tub or the toilet, cause that's not good, but other than that, she'd fall asleep on the counter."

Mario's words were a little confusing; however, Charles said, "No, that's not good."

Mario replied, "Cause I think it's probably like one of those things where it's like you're fine until you're not, and you don't know that you're, (Pause in his words) she's trying to do stuff, but she can't. She doesn't know that because it's like it just starts to kick in. You know, I don't know how that stuff works. She's trying to do her normal stuff. Doing the dishes, cleaning, and cooking. One time, she fell asleep on the counter with a knife in her hand, trying to cook. I would be like, 'man, give me that.'"

Mario and Charles laughed even though they knew it wasn't a funny matter.

Mario said to Charles, "It's a good thing she knew that I knew how to cook, so she would go, here you go."

Charles asked, "You mean she didn't get angry with you?"

Mario said, "No, not with cooking."

Taking Care of Bree and Boxer

Charles said, "I know Bree and Boxer must have been off the hook when your mom wasn't there, especially since your mom wasn't there to correct or yell at them when they were doing something wrong, because man, your mom can do some yelling to get them to do what they need or are supposed to do. I remember you telling me that sometimes your mom would be gone for a month at a time."

Mario let out a sigh, "I don't remember, I don't remember a lot of things. I mean, I don't remember the specific details of what me and the kids were doing. I remember what I was doing outside and what I was doing when I came home. I don't know, Bree and Boxer weren't that difficult. I mean, because back then they were too young, like, I would make them clean up and stuff, so I would make sure they ate and cleaned themselves and brushed their teeth, that's it. They just watched TV, went outside, and played, just like normal kids do. It would have been more difficult for them, but they had each other.

Like I said, they watched TV together and played together. If it was just one kid, you had to pay attention to that one kid. I helped them with their homework, but most of the time they didn't have homework because they were like in first grade, kindergarten."

Life Goes On

Charles could hear Mario's mom still crying and moaning in pain. He just felt as if he needed to do something, but at the same time, he didn't want to disrupt the family's normal routines that had worked for them over the years. Everyone was walking around as if this was normal. Every now and then, Charles would hear Boxer say, "Mommy, are you okay?" Mena would say, "I'll be alright."

Then Charles would hear Boxer go back into his room to play on his PS5. Bree was busy talking on her cellphone to her friends, ignoring her mother completely putting on makeup and fake eyelashes. Amelia was busy packing a suitcase for her mom, just in case she had to stay at the hospital. Amelia had no words to say to her mom. She followed her mom's directions to get this and get that. Then she would go back to typing something on her laptop for school.

Mario's stomach started to bubble. He was all of a sudden hungry. He said to Charlie, "Hey, man, do you want some delicious potato soup that my Mum Mum made? It's the best in town."

Charles felt guilty for saying yes, ignoring the facts of life going on in the house, but his stomach won over, and he said, "Sure."

Mario then said, "I just want to make sure you're not hungry or starving like we were from time to time. Not having much food in the house didn't happen until my mom went to the hospital. It also happened when my stepdad and mom separated. Amelia and I would eat very little. There wasn't much food left over. Sometimes it would come right down to us splitting a hashbrown."

Mario said, "Man, I'm hungry. I don't know. The last thing I'm going to say about this is that I think it would have affected me more if I was, uh, let's see how I should put this? I don't want to say I'm not compassionate, but when people are crying and stuff, I don't know what to do, I just say you can go over there."

Charlie was very confused about that statement, but didn't ask Mario to explain it. He just let Mario continue on.

Mario went on talking, "You're not getting any pats on the back. You're not getting any hugs from me. Like, what do you want? Like I don't, I don't, I don't know. I've always been like that. If it's close family I care about, but even if you are my family, if you're not in the circle, I don't care. Some people in my family are not in my circle, so if something happens to them, nothing will change in my life. I don't want anything to happen to them, but if it does, I would be like…"

Mario just shook his shoulders and continued with what he was saying, "Funny, like you know when people come over, and they say you should do something? I'm like, no! No, just sit here and relax."

Charles began to think this was not a normal family. How could he relax when all he was hearing was the pain of agony? He felt weird with Mena being in pain and crying, and barely walking around. Mario knew that his mom was strong, and she would curse, curse, curse, and he would say she'd be alright. If he knew that his mom was a weak person, then he would have helped and been around more.

Denver, Colorado

Out of the sky, blue Mario began to think about when he was younger. He remembered when they lived in Colorado. It was the worst place their family could have lived in for his mom, as far as he was concerned. The climate was cold and elevated. Mario knew from reading books that Denver Colorado has a negative impact on those with Sickle Cell. The elevation is too high. Denver Colorado was perched a mile above sea level, at 6,800 feet. Mena had to stay hydrated and avoid extreme exercise. The elevation was just too high. It caused a lot of breathing problems for his mom. Mario only knew that his mom was in the hospital again, and again, and again; however, she would always return strong. She mostly complained about her stay. That was one of the reasons why they left Colorado. Mario knew that it was all about stress, for he had heard the doctor say that the reason his mom was in so many crises was because of stress. The relationship with his stepdad was more stressful than Colorado itself.

Mario thought in his head, "Rex was doing too much. He was doing all types of stuff. Since their separation, Mena has not been in the hospital that often. Instead of once or twice a month, it is now 4 or 5 times a year.

Conversation Ending

"Hey!" Mario said, "Okay, enough of this talk, let's go play on my PS4. It's my first game console I bought with my money." Mario said happily, "And guess what? I still have it! Two hundred and twenty dollars. I would get off work on payday, get something to eat, and then I would wait for Chris, my uncle, to get home every Friday. Chris and I would go to the mall. I had a consistent job, my first. I was still a teenager, and I had never had that kind of money before. I didn't pay rent or anything. All I was asked to do was to get water and milk. I was like Okay! Which I don't think I even did that consistently. I think I resorted to giving Pup Pup my grandfather twenty dollars a week. I didn't remember to do that because I didn't have a car. Mostly, Bree plays it now. Boxer has a PS5. I play it when he's in school. I grew up with video games, but not like Bree and Boxer. Hey, I changed my mind. Boxer is leaving. Let's go play his PS5 in his room. It will take your mind off my mom."

Chapter 10

We Have to Let You Go
(Autumn Leaf)

Autumn Leaf takes on many colors—Yellow, orange, red, and brown. Autumn leaves are very beautiful and vibrant. Sometimes Autumn is called Fall. Both have their ups and downs in popularity. In the U.S., it's Fall. In Britain, it's Autumn. Their hormones within the plant are activated to begin the abscission process—(separation of leaves from plants at a special separation layer). The process has 3 steps: resorption, protective layer formation, and detachment.) Wikipedia, Dictionary.com, https://www.merriam-webster.com

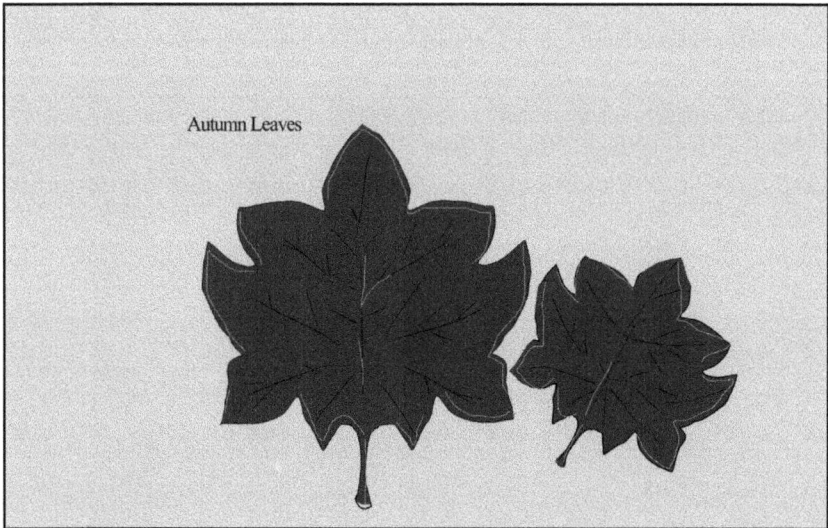

Autumn Leaves

Phone Call Interruption

Lisa was enjoying her quiet day off from work when her cell phone rang. She looked down and saw that it was her niece, Autumn, calling. Lisa wondered what Autumn could be calling about. Most of the time, when Autumn would call, it was always something dramatic or some crisis she was going through. Most of the time, it would be Autumn complaining about something that was happening at her job. Lisa thought to herself, *should she answer it or let Autumn leave a message?* Lisa and her niece were remarkably close, but Autumn's phone calls were usually long, and she spoke at the speed of lightning, which drove Lisa insane trying to keep up with what Autumn was saying. Since the passing of Lisa's mother, her close relatives have always called on Lisa for advice. Lisa had given Autumn advice from time to time about everything and anything. Lisa loved Autumn's name because it represented the beauty of all colors. It truly was a beautiful autumn day. The leaves were falling, the wind was brisk, and the air was cool. What a perfect setting! Through the thrill of it all, there was going to be work to do later, such as raking up all those leaves in her yard. The branches and pine needles were already falling to the ground; however, Lisa didn't want to think about that right now. She just wanted to enjoy every moment of the day, and yet her husband, Bruce, was calling her before he went on with his chores for the day. All Lisa wanted was a day to herself doing what she wanted to do. Bruce's morning sleep was cut too short, so Lisa's me time was fading away with the interruption of her husband and niece.

Autumn had grown up to be a beautiful young lady. She was very intellectual and was determined to make it on her own. The only thing that was getting in her way was her Sickle Cell Anemia. Just when she felt as if she were taking two steps forward, she would be knocked two feet backwards and then some by this infectious disease.

Lisa decided to pick up the phone to find out what it was that Autumn wanted to talk about. She started off by saying, "Auntie!"

What Started Out As A Picture-Perfect Day

Autumn was on her way to work. She traveled down a beautiful tree-lined road. Some days, when it was foggy, the fog would look like a lace curtain gracefully going back and forth across the road. It was 6:00 a.m. It was a picture-perfect day that brought happiness to Autumn's heart and mind. The drive to work was well worth it. How could this not turn into a beautiful day when she saw the splendor of God's love everywhere?

Autumn parked her car, and she was ready to do what she loved best: making her customers happy. No sooner had Autumn placed her things down than her boss, Nicki, approached her. Nicki's name was quite fitting for her. Nicki means the one who wins overall. She was always right in everything she did. No one could win an argument with her. Nicki called Autumn to come into the back room.

Nicki didn't wait to quickly blurt out the words: "Autumn, I'm glad you're here early. We need to talk."

That lovely day in Autumn's mind seemed to start to fade away before it even started.

Nicki proceeded to say, "You have been a great asset to our company. I need to give you a short evaluation. Have a seat."

Autumn thought to herself, "Okay, maybe it's going to be an enjoyable day. I'm a great asset to the company and impressive to my customers."

Autumn wasn't expecting an evaluation. She had arrived at work early so that she could have a little time for herself, her me time, and finish her green tea and donut.

Nicki said, "I know what you're thinking. Oh, don't worry, I will let you take an early break so that you can have your, what did you always call it? Your me time." Autumn had stolen that line from her Aunt Lisa.

"Your evaluation will be scaled 0-5. Okay, here we go! You are always on time for work, a 5, and your manners are excellent, a 5. You are overly mannerly. Your customer service is a 5. You are always greeting your customers with a polite hello and welcoming them to our shoe store. Your sales definitely meet our expectations. Your motto is "sell in 3's." You are our best retailer in helping customers open a new credit card account, which earns a 5. Your organization is a 5. You are such a smooth and quick operator in stocking our apparel and shoes in our store. When asked to work overtime, you are always on board a 5. I am so grateful for that."

Autumn was boiling over with joy at this evaluation. She said to herself, *"It's going to be a lovely day. I am knocking this evaluation out of the park."*

That's a phrase her mother, Phyllis, would use all the time. Autumn's mother's name means helping to keep the baby young. Autumn always felt that was just what her mother was trying to do. Keep her young and treat her like a baby. Keeping the young part, Autumn didn't mind, but the baby part of it had to go. She was now a grown woman.

Nicki continued, "You almost have a perfect score except for one thing."

Autumn looked her boss, Nicki, straight in the eye and said, "What is it?"

Nicki answered her directly, "It's your attendance that is a 2. This is causing a real problem for me. I can't depend on you to be here when you are scheduled. When you're out, it's not just a day. It could be a week or two weeks. Honestly, sometimes I'm afraid to even put you on the schedule. I'm afraid that after this week, I am going to have to let you go."

Autumn's heart dropped. Autumn was traumatically saddened by the words that had just come out of her boss's mouth. This would completely change her life, her goals, and her dreams with this company. She wanted to become a manager someday so badly. She knew all the ins and outs of this company. Stress was overtaking her body as her Sickled Cells did. Her Sickle Cells prevent her from living the life she was trying to manage. Her heart began to race. She felt as if she could hear her heartbeat pounding out of harmony. This was truly one of the heavy moments in her life. She could not and would not return home to live with her mother. She was finally making it on her own. Autumn was so overwhelmed about leaving the company she loved, so much so that she could hardly breathe.

Autumn burst out in anger, "How could you let me go, because I know that I am your best employee. I can't help it if my body goes into a Sickle Cell Crisis. I have no control over that. I never know from day to day or how long the crisis is going to last. The main thing I know is that I was born with it. It causes me fatigue, anemia, pain episodes, and bone problems. All I can do is listen to my body. I cannot dismiss what my body is telling me to do. I have to be alert to the warning signs of my body at all times. When my body calls for rest, I rest. When I need an IV treatment to help move the cells through my body, I try not to delay. If I seek treatment early, I can try to keep my symptoms under control. There have been many times I have sacrificed and worked through my pain knowing that I needed treatment."

Nicki said, "That's the point; you're unpredictable. I don't know from day to day if you're going to be here."

Autumn felt paralyzed, and her lips were shimmering. Finally, her body felt like Autumn leaves that are not simply blown off a tree but are separated from the tree in a highly controlled process before they fall. Autumn felt as if her flesh was changing color with all the emotions her body was going through. She was going through the three stages, just like Autumn leaves. First, she could feel the absorption and circulation of her cells and tissue, which made her feel the pain of dissolving bone in her arm and shoulder, and her skin turning blue, just like the autumn colors. Secondly, she had lost the ability to be outspoken to save her job. She no longer felt the protection of her rights as an employee, like the roots of a tree no longer protecting the leaves with nourishment. Finally, she felt like a failure. She was dying inside. Just as leaves falling from a tree. She was now detached from a job.

Autumn felt as though she needed to provide an even deeper explanation of what had happened to her. Autumn said, "I explained this all to you before. My Sickle Cells jam inside my body and my whole cells can't flow to give my lungs, heart, and brain the oxygen I need to live. I have worked for this company for 6 years, and I have probably called out at least 15 times."

Nicki said, "Yes, that's true; however, you have called out at least once every month this year. This is detrimental to me and the other employees. They either can or can't come in to take your place, or they have to pick up the load when you're not here. Then, I have to revamp my schedule over and over again. I can't find employees to cover your shift for days and weeks. I'm afraid I have to let you go."

Autumn thought to herself. *"I am going to have to investigate this matter. What are my rights as an employee, especially with the impressive evaluation I just had? I will start by calling my Aunt Lisa."*

She knew her Aunt had always given her great advice in so many ways. Then she would turn to her cousin, Mena. She would speak with her mother later when she could figure out some things on her own. Hopefully, her mother, Phyllis, would be proud of her.

The Falling Of The Leaves

Driving back to her home, Autumn began to drift off deeply in thought, looking at the leaves on the trees. Her major in college was Biology, the study of life. She loved the study of nature. She said to herself, *"I am so glad my mom named me Autumn because that was the perfect name for me. Green leaves, the leaves are bright green in the summer. The grass and leaves are growing so fresh. I've heard the saying that when you say someone is green, it means they have little experience in life or even in a particular job. I had the perfect job. Now, as far as little experience in life, that was me. I have always depended on my mother for everything since I was a baby. I felt brand new and innocent. Even as a teenager, I still had little experience in life. I began to have trouble expressing my feelings. I would just be quiet and let others express their feelings and thoughts, just looking pitiful. Then the feeling of depression and stress would just take over my whole body. So, I ended up in the hospital, filled with pain and agony. My mother would always be at my side day and night. Sometimes I felt extremely bad because I knew that she had to take off work to comfort and protect me from any bad decisions that I felt I might make, regarding my health care. I don't mind talking to myself when I am driving because it's such a long and lonely drive back home. I glanced at the Red leaves that appear because the nights are too cold for the sugars to move downward in the tree. In bright light, the sugars become trapped in the leaves, forming the red pigments. The reddish-colored leaves stunt growth, and poor flowering is a common symptom of nitrogen, magnesium, or potassium deficiency. It's an attraction to the human eye. Wow! That sounds just like my body. I'm attractive, if I may say so myself, and I have a mineral deficiency.*

Having Sickle Cell has stunted my growth. The cells get trapped in my veins, especially when it's cold. I should have been a scientist with all this knowledge that I remember. High school taught me Biology well. Red can symbolize passion, strength, and love. When I display these qualities, I attract more people to me, just like the red leaves. The doctors and nurses are so much nicer. I receive more compliments when I wear red; however, the color red can sometimes be perceived as dangerous and poisonous. It brings on anger. A red flag is the best way to describe it. It conveys danger. It can bring out so many emotions and feelings. My blood pressure can go up or down, my metabolism can increase or slow down, my heart rate can beat out of control, and it can be followed by my respiration increasing.

Now, Orange leaves catch my eyes. Have you ever seen an orange highway sign? It says uneven pavement; it alerts you to possible dangers. The leaves are extremely close to falling off. Deficiency is infinite. That's the way the blood cells work in my body. The blood cells are not equal. The Sickle Cells outnumber my whole cells. My body tells me I need maintenance on my body. This alert makes me extremely tired. I have severe iron deficiency, swelling in my hands and feet, shortness of breath, irregular heartbeat, and dizziness. Lord, please don't let me get dizzy while I am driving.

The radiance of the yellow leaves heightens my moment. This is where I am in my life. Yellow symbolizes intellectual thoughts, creativity, happiness, and the power of persuasion. I don't need anyone to persuade me to do things that I don't want to do. I am mature now, and I can see clarity in many things. My family no longer influences me in making decisions. I am grown, and now, at the age of 26, I can ask their opinions about things, but when it comes down to it, I can decide by analyzing everything that may affect my health. My way of living. I own victory in my life. I can decide which direction to go. I can deal with situations with my mind, not my heart. No one can any longer get over on me. It may sound crazy to me, talking to myself and answering myself, but I know that I'm not crazy. I have the power to persuade myself to be happy and to utilize my creativity through journal writing.

Now, here comes Brown leaves. My heart is saddened by all the brown leaves that have fallen to the ground. When I think about it, brown is a combination of orange and black. You can also combine red, yellow, and black to make brown. I think to myself, 'How do you know all this?' It's because I love art. I used to use the color wheel all the time. Brown can signify the earth in my mind. The place that I am headed, however, I am determined to beat the odds in living past 50. It makes me think of diverse cultures. People are almond, beige, bisque, mocha, and chocolate, ranging from cool to warm browns, and from light to dark. Auburn is my favorite because it is reddish brown. It makes me happy. There are wonderful shades of brown out there in this world for everyone to see. It reminds me that Sickle Cell doesn't discriminate based on the color you are. It's not prejudice. Someday, I'm afraid that I may become bisque, which is a pale, creamy shade of brown. That's when life seems to fade away from me.

What a murky sight to see! Purple-Black Leaves. They are overpowered by the green chlorophyll, making the leaves look black. I loved biology as much as I loved art. You can see a gleam of purple shining through in the sunlight."

Autumn could recall seeing the black blotches on the leaves at some point in time. Taking an early morning walk, sadness seemed to cover her every waking moment.

She said, out loud to herself, "Some bacteria, due to the weather conditions, had caused a disease to slowly creep into the leaf itself. The roots began to suffocate in wet conditions. The cause was root rot and fungal infections, which resulted from the plant being waterlogged. What a good science memory I have. Just like sickle cell disease that has crept slowly into my body, as I age, slowly suffocating my whole good cells out."

Autumn read somewhere that there are 134 shades of black. Suddenly, sadness crept into Autumn's heart and mind, for she knew that the changes in the leaves from green to orange, to yellow, to brown, and finally to purple-black meant the leaves were coming to their end. Autumn whispered, "Black has beautiful names such as ebony, jade, spider, sable, midnight, onyx, charcoal, and the list goes on."

Autumn knew that black was the darkest color on this planet. It was a mystical color. Autumn blurted out, "It can make me elegant, sophisticated, powerful, and strengthen me to have authority in situations when needed. Yet at the same time, it can bring on a feeling of fear, depression, grief, and mourning. It could mean evil and death for me."

Many times, her energy and strength were taken away from her. She fears dying at an early age. Autumn thought again and again to herself. In a strong voice, Autumn elaborated in detail, "The hospital doesn't make me feel elegant or sophisticated, and yet there are times when I do feel powerful and filled with positive and negative energy. I can control what the doctors and nurses do to me, and I can advocate for myself and others in my cold, dreadful room. That brings neutrality between us all." Autumn took a deep breath, "I hope I did a decent job at recording myself. I will put this in my journal when I get home. Journal writing makes my day. See, I'm not crazy after all."

Autumn finally made it home and just sat in the parking lot, crying for a moment as she looked at and observed the leaves, her destiny.

Autumn recorded again in solemn sadness, "Darkness has been simmering in my bones all my life, and it will until the final destiny of death has been accomplished, just like the fallen leaves of various hues. They have taken their rest in beauty, covering Mother Earth, and so will my body, as my ashes are spread among the earth.

Autumn finally arrived home, but before she began to write in her journal entry, "Dear Journal," she thought she would call her Aunt Lisa first to get some advice about her Job. Autumn said, "Yes, my Auntie will know what to do. She'll give me some great advice."

Chapter 11

Journal Writing (Fossils)

Fossils—the preserved remains of plants and animals whose bodies were buried in sediments, such as sand and mud, under ancient seas, lakes, and rivers. Fossils also include any preserved trace of life that is typically more than 10,000 years old. Soft body parts decay soon after death, but the hard parts, such as bones, shells, and teeth, can be replaced by minerals that harden into rock. In very exceptional cases, soft parts like feathers, plant ferns, or other evidence of life, such as footprints or dung, may also be preserved. https://www.bgs.ac.uk

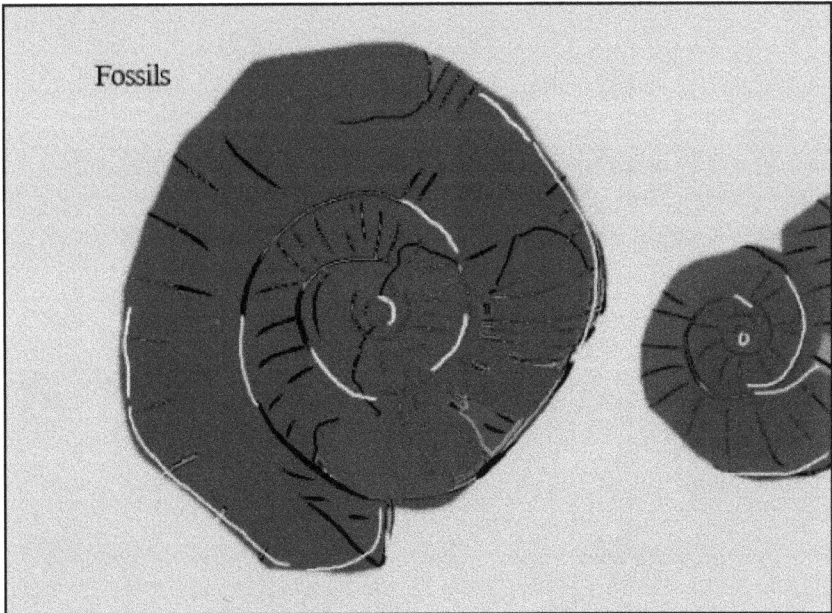

Fossils

Autumn knew that someday she would pass away, most likely at an early age. She knew that she hadn't accomplished anything in life that the world would remember, so she took a course in Journal writing with Bee. She knew that her bones wouldn't amount to anything, and they wouldn't be preserved like fossils. She knew that her soft skin would start decaying as organic matter, and the maggots would feed on her dead tissue. So, what was there left to do but to leave some sort of writing that would be like a footprint that hardens in the sand? She would process a recording of her thoughts each day.

Preserve Writings

She would start by saying, "Dear Feelings." She would begin with the words of her mother, Phyllis, about what she was like when she was an infant until the day she could remember. Her mother's perfect name, Phyllis, also meant foliage. It meant a collective leafy canopy of trees. Her mom was always covering her, almost smothering her at times. She was now twenty-seven years old. All her life, people were telling her what she could and couldn't do. In her journal writing, no one could tell her what to say or do. It would be a combination of a diary and a journal. She felt that she would be expressing her daily experiences, as well as her thoughts and observations about all things in life, and every idea that she might have. Hopefully, someone would preserve her writings, and the world would be so much kinder and warmer to those with Sickle Cell. She would especially dedicate her writing to her mother, Phyllis, and cousin, Mena. Phyllis and Mena knew what she was going through. Her journal recording would begin with her recording herself using her cell phone.

Three-Four Months Old

She decided to record her mother Phyllis' words. She would write them in her journal later. She asked her mother to start talking.

Phyllis begins by saying, "They told me that they knew that you had Sickle Cell before you were born when they did a test on me. They figured it out while you were in my stomach. Your first crisis you were only three or four months old. You had swollen hands and swollen legs, and you cried. I thought you had gotten bitten by a bee, but that couldn't have been true because it was the month of December. I said to myself, 'It's wintertime.' Your hands and your legs were two sizes big, and you cried. I just kept rubbing you and rubbing you. I took a warm towel and placed it on your face, then continued to cuddle you, and you finally fell asleep. The towel is now called Oaky. Which you still have to this day. You had to take penicillin from day one until you were twelve. Finally, I told them that they wouldn't give you any more because your body must be immune to it by now. It can't be helped. That was the only medicine that you were on.

When you were two years old, you wouldn't walk because you were in so much pain. I had to hold you for a week and a half, and you would not walk."

Autumn interrupted, "Wow! You really had to carry me?"

Phyllis said, "Yes, you wouldn't walk on your feet, you wouldn't use your hands. You were in just so much pain, and your eyes became yellow. First of all, you were born with jaundice. Your eyes look lime green and yellowish, so many people thought that you were blind. You were now about two years old, and the doctors said that it wasn't yet affecting your liver. At the age of two years old, that's when the Sickle Cell started really bothering you a lot. Like I said, it started when you were three or four months old, and your limbs would swell, and you would cry, and then down the road, I guess it got worse when you were three. Your legs hurt, and you would cry. I would have to pat you down. I put ice on you."

Autumn spoke in a thrilling voice and said, "What you put ice on me? That was one of the worst things you could have done."

Phyllis replied, "I know, right? The doctors recommended it. It depended on what kind of pain you were in. It was to cool it down. You know how you are; it's almost like when you have a charley horse - they tell you to heat it up and then they tell you to cool it down. It was like that."

Autumn replied, "Mom, that was an old remedy. That's not something that they would recommend right now."

Phyllis said, "Yea, back then they told me to put cold packs where you were paining and then I would use hot packs to get the blood flowing."

Autumn said, "Mom, that's crazy."

Phyllis' facial expression looked as if she was disappointed in herself.

Phyllis replied, "I know, but that's how it was."

"That reminds me of a time when you were left at home with your brother, who was nine, and you went into a crisis. We lived on an Indian Reservation. You couldn't walk, and I was at work. Scout took you on his back, along with Tai Tai the dog, to your grandmother's house, which was about half a mile away. Your grandmother, Ann, called me at work to ask what she should do. I told her to take you to the hospital immediately."

Phyllis began to speak about other treatments that she thought would work and went on explaining, "I would take a towel and put it in the microwave just enough so that you could stand the temperature. I would lay it on you so that your blood would start flowing."

Autumn said, "I am so glad that times have changed; they were just making things worse for Sickle Cell patients, making our blood jam even more."

Phyllis didn't reply to Autumn's statement about saying I'm glad times have changed, for she was too busy thinking about other things that happened to Autumn, so Phyllis continued talking:

"You didn't have any diets, but you used to eat powder. I asked the doctors why you ate powder, and they said that's one of the crises you have. I mean, like your cousin, Mena, she ate soap. That's something you guys did, that's what you craved."

Autumn said, "That's ridiculous, I'm sure that didn't have anything to do with having Sickle Cell. Those doctors didn't know what to say; people in general just crave wacky things. Like eating toilet paper, smelling gas, smelling fabric softener, and the list can go on and on, yet they don't have Sickle Cell."

Phyllis giggled and said, "You still have the recording going?"

Autumn said, "Yes."

Five or Six Years Old

Phyllis said, "Okay, when you were about five or six years old, we were on our way to North Carolina. You became very dehydrated. You used about a week's worth of underwear and two bags of pull-ups. We went to the hospital in North Carolina. They said that they didn't have a pediatrician, so they had to transfer you to another hospital, which was an hour away. They wouldn't let me ride with you to the hospital in the ambulance because of insurance reasons. So, I'm crying again. I've only cried about three times since you've been born. I cried because they were strangers, and you didn't know them, and I couldn't go. So, we followed them, and when we got there, one of the Social Service women there asked if I had abused you, and I said, 'Ma'am, I live in Salisbury. We are about four or five hours away from home. I did not come this far to abuse my child. You need to check her records. You need to call the hospital and see why my daughter is the way she is. She's dehydrated, and she is having a crisis, and she needs help. Do not come into my room anymore.' The Social Service woman looked at me and said, 'I'm sorry.'

I said, just because we're black, just because we are traveling doesn't mean that I am abusing my daughter. I don't know what other people do, but I love my daughter. I take care of my daughter. So, she walked out, and to make up for it, she sent a clown into the room. You looked at the clown, Autumn, and said, 'Get out! I don't like clowns.' I said, 'Autumn.' You said, 'Mommy, he's not funny, I'm in pain, and I don't feel like this right now.' So, Autumn, you said to the clown, 'Please leave.' So, the clown left. He never came back to the room. I asked them to transfer us to the University of Maryland so that I could be closer to you, and that was where your doctors are. He had one phone to each ear. On one phone, the doctor explained to my insurance company that they needed an ambulance because the helicopter was broken and that I needed to go to the University of Maryland. On the other phone, he was also talking to my captain at work because I told the doctor that I was going to be fired and that I was on probation. The doctor explained to him that this child is sick. She needs to go to the University of Maryland Hospital. She's at the hospital right now. Please don't fire her. So, he told the doctor to give me the phone. I was about to have a panic attack. I was like 'Captain, I'm in North Carolina. My daughter is in the hospital.'

My captain said, 'Calm down, calm down. You're not going to get fired. You have a legit reason. You're in the hospital, your daughter is in the hospital.'"

Phyllis went on to explain, "So, to make a long story short, they took us both by ambulance. Joe, your dad, and Scout, your brother, left, and by the time they got home, Scout went straight to school."

Scout's name was quite fitting for him. It means to listen or someone who gathers information. Missing school was not an option for Scout. He didn't want to miss any information that was going to be on the test the next day. He was about fifteen.

Joe, Autumn's father's name means (God Will Give). How fitting Phyllis felt that he had given her a precious daughter she adored so much!

Phyllis' last words about that trip were, "Interestingly, on the way to the hospital, the ambulance stopped at McDonald's for you because you said, 'I'm hungry.' When we arrived in Baltimore, we stayed there for a week."

Now, when you were about four and a half, you asked me if you were going to die."

Autumn asked, "I said that?"

Phyllis said, "Yes, Autumn, you said, 'Am I going to die because the pain hurt so bad?' and I said, 'God's got you in His hands; You will be alright.' So just like when you were two years old, now four, I would still take and rub you and always massage you. I would rub you down and rub you down. I would put pain medicine on you and just keep rubbing you down. You would always have like Auh, the crisis would be in your shoulders and in your legs, so I mostly rubbed your legs. There wasn't too much I could do about your shoulders."

Elementary School

Phillis said, "Now, when you started elementary school, you missed quite a bit of time in school. I still always made you do your homework.

The teachers told me that you didn't have to. You were out like two weeks at a time, three weeks at a time."

Autumn said, "I know Mommy and I would always ask you why I had to do my homework, and you would say, I don't want you to fall behind in school. Your hands aren't broke."

Phillis kept talking, "You might be in pain some days; however, some days you would feel okay. Some days you could do your homework. You weren't going to just lie in this bed and not learn. Some days, the pain wasn't so bad when you couldn't do your homework. I repeat, like I said, your hands weren't broke. You were hooked up to an IV in the hospital, so what else could you do but lie there? I would go to your school often to get your homework, or they would give it to your cousin Leo."

Leo's name means Lion. That is just what he looked like. He grew hair all around his face and on the top of his head. He wasn't afraid of anything. His mom could always count on him for anything. That would include the whole Wright family, and he could well count on him. Leo was always dependable. Phyllis always looked forward to Leo bringing Autumn her homework.

Phillis told Autumn, "Sometimes the teachers would give him the homework, and sometimes they wouldn't. They would say, 'Oh, it's okay; she doesn't have to worry about it, and I would say yes, she does.'"

Autumn would ask, "I can't really remember, but what about your job? How could you work if you were in the hospital with me?"

Seven Years Old

Phyllis had no problem answering that question. "Well, if you were at the hospital in our area here, I would go to work, at night, from eleven to seven, and then after work, I would go to the hospital and spend time with you all day. If I fell asleep when it was time for me to leave for work, the nurses would wake me up. When I would go out of town to Johns Hopkins or the University of Maryland, I would take time off, and I would just stay up there for a week. When I came home, your Aunt Lisa, or your grandmom, Ann, would watch you so that I could go to work. The doctors and nurses treated you like a queen; they loved you. Whatever you wanted, you would get even though you were mean."

Autumn replied, "Well, Mommy, I was in so much pain."

"When you were about seven years old, you had a crisis, and they tried to give you a needle, but you kicked the nurse. So, they put you in a straitjacket. I was crying and you were crying, and your dad, Joe, was looking at me and he was like, 'Phyllis, it's all right.' I was like, 'No, she's too young; they shouldn't be putting a straitjacket on her, that's for crazy people.' Joe replied, 'Well, she kicked the nurse.' Autumn, you shouted, 'How would you like to be stuck with a needle ten or fifteen times? Let me stick you, you give me the needle, and I will stick you.' That's what you said to the nurse, and they just looked at you and said, 'Bless her heart.' They gave you another needle, they took blood and gave you the IV because at first you wouldn't let the nurse do it, and I finally said, 'Autumn, let me tell you something, when you are mean to these nurses, they will take their time giving you medicine, they will take their time coming to see you. I said you need to change your attitude. I said, it's not going to work when you are being mean to them. You already have one cousin that's like that, Mena. I said, for you to be like that, I'm telling you, it's not going to work, and I'm not going to let you treat them like that. I said, because I'm here every day. I see what they do to you every day. I am with you every day. I always stayed at the hospital, even as I said, when you would go to Johns Hopkins in Baltimore, I went, so I knew what they were doing to you."

Nine or Ten Years Old

"Now, when you were nine or ten, the teachers came and gave you gifts. When I was playing softball, the team gave me two hundred and fifty dollars to buy you some gifts. I thank them for supporting you. The whole team always supported you and looked out for you. They would take turns watching you at the games, making sure you weren't in pain. You didn't go to too many of my games, probably only about five. It was either too hot or too cold. One thing that you would do is always ask questions. What is that for? What is this? What is that? You knew what type of needles they should use. You know what kind of medication you should take. You told them that you were allergic to the plastic tape; you knew everything about yourself if they didn't know. They said that you were very smart and very bright. You told them 'Yea, because some of these nurses don't know what they are doing.' So, you knew everything that they did from the age of two until now."

Autumn wondered, "When I was young, do you remember the names of the medicines they were giving me?"

"No, Autumn, I don't really remember. It was just too many for me to remember. They wanted to give you Hydroxyurea. The side effects would be that your hair would fall out, your nails would turn yellow, and you could go blind. I said no. I asked, 'Is it USD approved?' and they said, 'Not yet.' It was like for cancer patients. I thought, 'No, my daughter is not getting that.' I never gave that to you ever."

Autumn asked, "Mommy, was my dad aware of whether or not he had Sickle Cell?"

Phyllis replied, "Well, you know some men don't get tested to see if they have the trait or not. Back then, nobody worried about that. If you liked somebody, you liked them. I knew that I had the Sickle Cell trait, but I never asked him if he had the trait. I didn't pay that any mind or attention. When the doctor found out that I was pregnant, he suggested that your father should get tested. So, I asked him, 'Do you have the trait or not?' and he said no. The doctor tested his blood, and he did have the Sickle Cell Trait. He didn't realize that he was born with it. He thought that you got the Sickle Cell trait somewhere later in life. After that, I had to go to the University of Maryland twice a month with you for nine months."

Autumn asked, "Well, mommy, how did you know that you had the trait?"

"Lisa told me that she had the Sickle Cell Trait, but that neither one of our parents knew who had the trait." Phyllis moved on to tell her story. "We were there so much, Autumn, that if you had to go to the bathroom. I knew how to unplug and plug the IV. I wouldn't let them give you a shower because I did it myself."

Phyllis had forgotten to tell Autumn something. Autumn would fix this later in her Journal writing. It was a good thing that she was recording her mother's words.

"Oh, I forgot to tell you that when you were probably about five, I think, and you had to have an emergency operation. They flew you from our hospital to the University of Maryland. You were hooked up to a machine. The machine was breathing for you for about two days. You had pneumonia. I was in there with you, and they told me that if you didn't walk or use the bathroom, you couldn't go home. Your dad said, 'Baby, if you're in pain, you don't have to walk or eat.'"

Phyllis said angrily, "Put him out." Phyllis turned and said to Joe, "The car is outside. Go home." Phyllis then said to him, "Autumn has to walk. She has to use the bathroom, and she has to eat." Phyllis turned to the nurse and said, "Nurse, he needs to leave. Please put him out." The nurse kindly asked him if he was willing to leave.

Autumn was shocked and asked, "Mommy, are you serious? You had the nurse put my daddy out?"

Phyllis replied, "Yep, Autumn, that's what I did. Joe knew from the beginning that you had to do all this. That you had to walk, eat, and poop before you could leave the hospital; it wasn't the first time. Like I said, you were about five years old then. He already knew this, but he was the type: if you didn't want to, you didn't have to. I would always make you do it. I would make you walk; make you get up and eat whether you wanted to do it or not."

Autumn said once again, "Mommy, I can't believe the nurse did that. He was my dad; she couldn't make him leave."

Phyllis said, "Oh, but she did. She put him out!"

Autumn then asked, "Well, how did we get home?"

Phyllis answered by saying, "My Uncle Clarence brought us home. His name means one who lives near the river, and he lived near a river when he was growing up and still does to this day. Uncle Clarence and his wife, Agnes, visit was short. Agnes' name means warm and kind-hearted. She would come and visit us every time we came to Baltimore. I truly appreciated it. They would bring us apples, oranges, and pears. I had lots of people come and visit us. A lady I met at a track meet would come and visit us."

Autumn was feeling grateful, "Mommy, I am glad you made me do all those things because I would have never done it."

Phyllis was now babbling all over the place with her stories. Phyllis continued, "Oh, and I would make you walk the floors, and you had a breathing tube, and I would make you use it even when you didn't want to. I would make you do everything that you didn't want to do. I would tell you to thank the nurse. I didn't care if you didn't like the food. I would make you eat some of it whether you liked it or not. I would massage you, but when you were really in pain, I would stop. Now that you are older, the doctors are treating you nicely, but they don't know anything. They don't know a thing. They will just be guesstimating. They're just trying to use different stuff. They really don't know. They gave you two blood transfusions while we were at the hospital."

Twenty-Seven Years Old

Autumn said, "Oh, mommy, even at my twenty-seven, they gave me a blood exchange that I didn't approve of. They waited until I was under medication, and I signed the papers. I was mad, and I was crying, and you were crying. It was my very first blood exchange."

Phyllis said, "I remember we both said no. I couldn't do or say anything because you were twenty-seven, so I couldn't do anything about it. You were half conscious and half not. You didn't know you were signing a paper for them to do the blood exchange. It left a mark in your throat, and you said that your throat was sore."

Autumn said, "Yeah, and I couldn't really talk. I'm sad that I have had to have two of them in my life; the second blood exchange was near my groin. I wouldn't let them put it in my throat again because it made my throat so sore. I could barely talk after that. I knew my friends couldn't come and see me at the hospital all the time, but it was nice that they came to see me at the house. Having company made me feel so much better. It made me feel less alone, and it made me realize that my family and friends cared. Some of my cousins were too young to come to the hospital anyway."

Make A Wish

Phyllis thought about a wonderful memory. Phyllis said, "Guess what, Autumn? I just finished watching the movie about the guy who started "Make a Wish." He is no longer the head of it, but he continues to support it. I was so glad that you had the opportunity to make a wish. I know that you wanted to meet the Rock, but going to the Mall of America for a shopping spree was best for you. You wanted a computer, and you wanted a phone, and I told you, Autumn, I can't buy you all that stuff."

Autumn said, "I remember. I was so mad with you that I had to make a choice. I really wanted to see the Rock."

Phyllis said, "I remember asking you, Do you really think that the Rock is going to give you his belt? Back then, I didn't really think that he would give you his belt. You were a total stranger and a kid that he didn't know. Wasn't the shopping spree worth it? You got twenty-five hundred dollars. You got to go see the Cincinnati baseball team play for free. You got a percentage off at every store we visited. You got to ride in a limousine to the airport from the house, and they flew you, me, and your brother, Scout, to Cincinnati for free. They paid for the hotel for four days. You got to stop at McDonald's. You also got to ride an indoor roller coaster, and everything you wanted, they gave to you. You are doing really well now. You have only been going to the hospital about two times a year. Remember, you almost went every month when you were younger. You stayed for weeks and weeks. It has gone down to a couple of days. I really can't say why it slowed down. I guess it's because you are older and stronger. You know how to manage your pain better. You know how to take care of yourself and fight through the pain. Now you can stand it a little bit longer before you have to go to the hospital. Your medications are stronger as well. You can take different kinds of medication that you couldn't when you were younger. You were limited to what you could have when you were a baby, and no more ice packs."

They both laughed. Autumn had a full ear for her mother's stories, so she thanked her so much for sharing her challenging moments from her life that she couldn't remember.

Autumn said, "This should be great, Mom, for me to write in my journal. I hope my fingers won't get cramped up from this long recording of your words. I better get busy writing in my journal."

Autumn hoped that this fossil writing of hers would last forever for the next generation. She had still planned on beating the odds. She would fight for longevity without pain! "Maybe my bones won't last forever, but maybe my words will."

Chapter 12

Relationships (Love Birds)

L ove Birds are social and affectionate. The name comes from the parrots' strong, monogamous pair bonding and the long periods that paired birds spend sitting together. https://en.wilkipedia.org

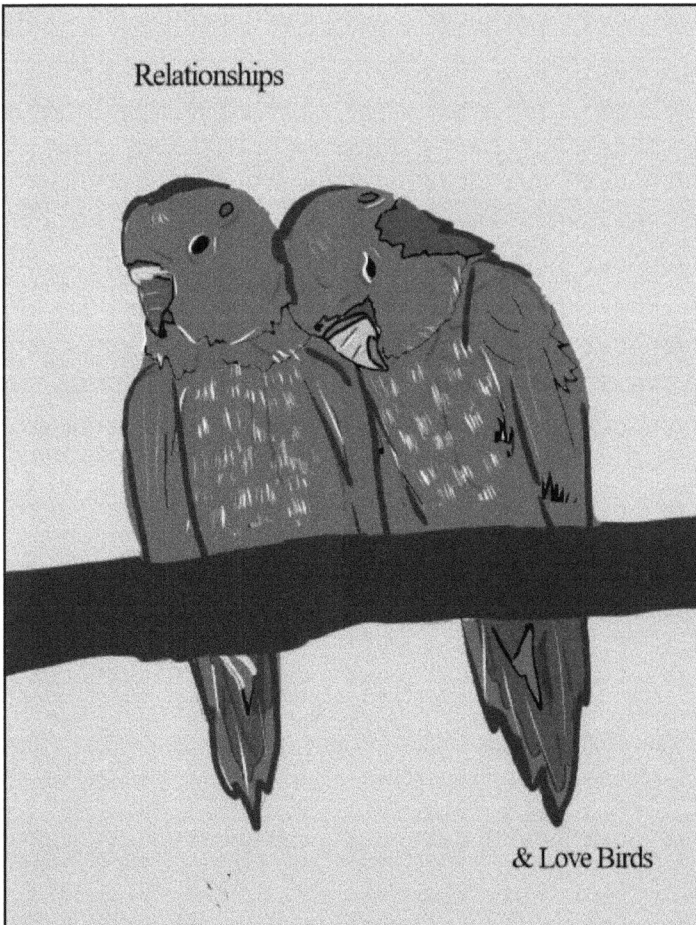

Relationships

& Love Birds

Back Down Memory Lane

Mena's relationships had been dwindling since Senior High School. She had been in a very toxic relationship with her son's father. His name is Keith, which means rigid and unyielding, just like the meaning of his name. They were not just compatible with one another, for they were both very temperamental. Their partnership was not a bonding relationship. They were intimate from time to time; their uncooperative behavior and mood pattern were the same. They were not compatible. They say opposites attract; well, this was not the case for them. Aggression can be easily aroused in love birds, and they do just that towards one another. They just couldn't see eye to eye on anything. Not even in the disciplining of their child. Having harmony in disciplining their child just went out the window. All Keith wanted was respect from his child. Sometimes, what a mother thinks is love can get in the way. Life was not easy for Mario, as he loved them both; however, Keith and Mena separated from one another and went their own way.

Mena's Mom once asked Mena's boyfriend, Keith, "Why do you treat women the way that you do?" He replied, "'Cause they let me."

Mena fell in love with a guy named Felipe, who was not just her lover but a friend. Felipe means a friend of horses. Felipe is the central character in Elizabeth Gilbert's book "Eat Pray Love." In the story, Felipe shows the protagonist what real love looks like. Felipe did just that in their relationship, but as time would have it, their relationship had become rocky. Felipe found himself home alone often. Mena was young at heart, going astray from time to time. He just wasn't good enough for her. One day, after the birth of their child, Amelia, Felipe just disappeared into thin air. Mena's family was extremely fond of him. They never knew the true story of why he left. To this day, they only have fond memories left of him.

Mena once found herself with someone who she felt would protect her and treat her special. He was in law enforcement. He was the worst of all her relationships. His name was Brutus. His name was associated with treachery if not cruelty. In English, it is sometimes used to express shock at betrayal by a friend or close associate. He was constantly loving someone else.

Marriage

Oh, happy day. One day, the phone rang, and it was Mena. "Mom, I'm getting married to a guy named Rex."

Rex means King. Springs from images of dinosaurs, a carnivorous predator. He thought he was king in trying to make people feel he was something he was not.

Mena said, "We will be moving out of the United States, and I was wondering if you could come to see us get married off. We are going to get married at the justice of peace tomorrow."

Lisa responded, "I haven't even met him yet. Are you sure you are ready for this?"

Mena answered, "Of course I am. His sister introduced us, and we have been dating for months. This is my opportunity to get far away from here."

Lisa was joyful and downhearted at the same time. She said, "But what about the kids?"

Mena responded, "I am taking all my children with me. I will be able to take care of them since Rex is a computer analyst. You should be happy for me. You will no longer have to be raising my kids for me. We plan to have kids of our own someday. He is accepting raising Mario and Amelia as well. I couldn't ask for more."

Mena and Rex did get married; however, the marriage was on a rollercoaster from the beginning. It had its ups and downs, but it was traumatic. From the start, they almost missed their wedding date that was scheduled at the courthouse. Mena had a habit of being late all the time, which was quite frustrating for Rex and the kids. She was so late that she didn't have the opportunity to get dressed for the wedding, even though her mom had bought her a beautiful dress with a flower arrangement. She got married in her torn jeans, but this didn't seem to bother Mena as long as the marriage took place.

The Argument

Eventually, Mena's sickness constantly interfered with life between Rex and the kids. "Rex, I need to go to the hospital. I just can't take this pain anymore. Can you take me?"

Rex replied, "I can't. I have a training course this morning, and I can't call out from work."

Mena shouted, "I don't give a darn about your job right now. I am in pain, and I can barely walk. If you don't take me, you're going to find that one day you're going to pay for all your so-called kingly decisions."

Mena began to say words that weren't found in the dictionary. They both exchanged unimaginable words with one another.

Boxer and Bree ran downstairs and said, "Mommy, daddy, stop yelling." Amelia slowly came down the steps as well.

Amelia said, "Mommy, the neighbors are going to hear you and Mr. Rex, and they'll call the police like the last time."

The vulgar language just spilled out of Mena's and Rex's mouths like nonstop lava. It ended with the hardening of their souls. Mena and Rex got to the point where there was no turning them around or trying to de-escalate them until they were ready to calm down or until one of them gave in. Pain always turned their Mom into someone they didn't know. Mena's back talk always made Rex pace the floor back and forth, along with smoking his cigarette. You would have thought he was sending out smoke signals for help. They were far from being love birds.

Love birds can form long-term relationships with people as well as other lovebirds. Mena never seemed to form any long-term relationships with any of her male friends. Mena and Rex couldn't seem to deal with themselves or the people around them, especially their neighbors. Mario never stepped foot downstairs, for he had become accustomed to their yelling and screaming. However, he knew that if Rex ever laid a hand on his mother, he would be forced to go into protection mode. He had done that before with his fleshly dad, Keith, when he tried to attack his mother. He was a warrior at heart when it came to his mother. Bree never forgot the last neighborhood they lived in; Mena and Rex were arguing and fighting with their neighbors. The police came and handcuffed both of them for disturbing the peace. Bree became so afraid that it was about to happen again to her parents.

The thought came into Bree's mind, "Who would raise them?"

Bree yelled, "Mommy, daddy, stop, the police will come and get you."

Boxer screamed, "You just let them try these hands; they are made for boxing. They will never take my mommy and daddy."

Amelia yelled at them, too, "Why do you guys always have to act the way you do? My friends' parents don't act like you guys do. I'm getting so tired of your fighting."

Rex walked out the door and drove off, spinning his car tires down the street. Mena began to cry even more because the pain was becoming like Charlie's horses all over her body. She couldn't walk any longer. Her legs felt as though they were descending into deep, quicksand. Her legs had become heavy as lead. It felt as though an anchor was attached to them, dragging behind her. Amelia ran next door for help from her mother's friend, Harmony. Her name means union. She was always trying to bring people together. Harmony could always help and intervene when Rex and Mena were no longer the lovebirds that she would see from time to time.

Harmony called for Mario to help her put his mother in the car. He did, and then she said to him, "Mario, help take care of the children," and off she went in a hurry to the hospital.

Amelia knew that Mario was only going to go back to his room, play on his game system, and ignore the kids until dinner time. Mario was a great cook, and he always made sure that his brothers and sisters ate, especially when there was a lot of food around the house to cook. When Rex would get paid, the family would go on a shopping spree and buy lots of groceries. The kids could get practically anything they wanted, and Mario would make their favorite dishes. This would only last a couple of weeks, and then the family was back to survival of the fittest. Living off of Kool-Aid, Pop-Tarts, hash browns, and peanut butter with jelly. Cereal was like a delicacy. Amelia, on the other hand, knew that she would be the babysitter for days, weeks, or maybe a month while her mother remained in the hospital. They all depended on Amelia until Mena returned from the hospital. Rex worked most of the time. There were times when he paid them no mind because he had said that he needed space of his own to gather himself from a hard day's work.

Moving Back Home

Amelia was hoping that her grandmother, Lisa, would come and rescue her once again. One day, that truly happened. Lisa came and took Amelia away. Lisa raised Amelia throughout her teenage years until one day Mena came back home with her family to live with her during the separation of their marriage. Lisa recalled the doctor saying one of the main factors inciting Mena's Sickle Cell Crisis was Mena's husband, Rex, causing her stress. When Mena moved back home with her mother, Lisa, she no longer seemed to go back and forth to the hospital constantly, and if she did go to the hospital, her stay was significantly shorter. The divorce had done them both some good. It would be another step in life that the children would have to get used to. By now, the kids had experienced friends coming and going throughout their lives. They were truly making new friends, but not keeping the old. When Mario and Amelia would try to reach out to their old friends, they had either moved away, changed the way they used to be, or had just forgotten them. Mario began to care less about having any friends at all. Amelia had a friend or two. She was very paranoid about certain people, and Mario stayed to himself. They had moved thirteen times, and they hadn't even graduated from high school yet. Bree and Boxer thought it was exciting to make new friends and move from place to place because they hadn't reached the point where best friends mattered. There would be no wanting to go to a dance or prom for Mario and Amelia, for they just didn't care anymore. Most teenagers have formed their circle of friends and best friends by now. Being the new kid on the block was not glorious at all. It only meant that people ignored you or tried to bully you. No one was going to mess with Mario, though, for he had the demeanor of 'try me and see what happens to you.' Mena always strayed away from the crowds, not talking to anyone or wanting to be a part of anyone or any crowd. Mario and Amelia were loners who stayed to themselves. Thank goodness they had cousins whom they could relate to, especially Mario. He had cousins almost his age on both sides of the family. He was special to both of his grandmothers. He was their first grandson, and even to this day, he remains special in their hearts.

Amelia hung out with her grandmother, Lisa, as much as she could because she knew that Lisa would always be there for her. This was not to say that her mother wouldn't, but Lisa's love was different. Amelia felt special around Lisa. Lisa did have other grandchildren that she loved from the heart. Ivy's children, Ashley and Tara, but that didn't matter. Amelia felt as if she was the only thing that mattered to her grandmother. Amelia loved the things her grandmother loved: 70s music, old movies, popcorn, and staying up late. They were always wiggling their mouths and noses at one another. This was their special gesture towards one another. This was the way they bonded. She understood what bonding was. It wasn't the bond that her parents had that didn't stick like glue.

Divorce

Reminiscing, Amelia finally recalled something that had been on her mind. Rex was sent away for a while because he had gotten into some deep trouble with the law. He was taken away from the family for about 4 years. Amelia thought this gave her mom time to heal and for them to rebuild their relationship with one another. It made room for them to grow close again. The day had come for Rex's release. They lacked sufficient evidence to keep him there, so they had to release him. Amelia wondered if she would lose the closeness she and her mom had formed again. Lo and behold, the fire that Mena and Rex had at the beginning was slowly going out. It was as if a blanket had covered the fire they used to have for one another, and the light got dimmer and dimmer. Finally, the fire they had for one another throughout the years was smothering out. Their love for one another became extinguished. The intense love they had for one another had no solid foundation. The harmony, trust, understanding, and communication they once had went up in smoke. It all ended in divorce. Amelia was relieved.

Mena remembered what her mother, Lisa, had told her. "Never let a man know how you truly feel. Never let him see you cry or see the pain in your heart."

Mena thought about those words throughout her relationship with Rex and all her relationships. She had given her heart away too many times. She had shed too many tears. Throughout all her relationships, they had forgotten about loving her. Her relationships only caused complications and stress.

Mena said to herself, "Why didn't I listen to my mother's advice? I'm going to depend on myself."

A Fresh Start In Life

Love Birds would be a figment of her imagination. She thought about her cousin, Natalie, Nota for short. Her favorite saying is, "For Real." Her name is linked to rebirth and fresh starts. Mena would do just that to have a fresh start in life. She would do fine by herself. Mena turned on her phone and played the song "All I Need" by Jennifer Hudson. The words couldn't have expressed her relationships with men any better. Mena had given away her heart too many times. She was no longer going to give herself away freely, as if to feel like she was cheapening herself. She was beginning to see that being all by herself wasn't that bad at all. She was done with the tears, pain, and sorrow that men had given her in anguish. She didn't want any memories of them echoing in her heart. She was looking for love that didn't love her back. Mena decided that she would turn her focus back on herself. Her new beginning in life would be "It's all about me." She would start by loving herself. She would be her strength and confidence. She would no longer stand against the wall. She would no longer be put in a bad situation or be forced to do something that she didn't want to do. There would be no love bird connection here. She would no longer entertain the thought of lovebirds needing attention and affection. Mena thought about lovebirds described as being in a honeymoon phase of their relationship. Well, that would no longer exist, not for a long time with anyone.

Mena recited her poem to Natalie.

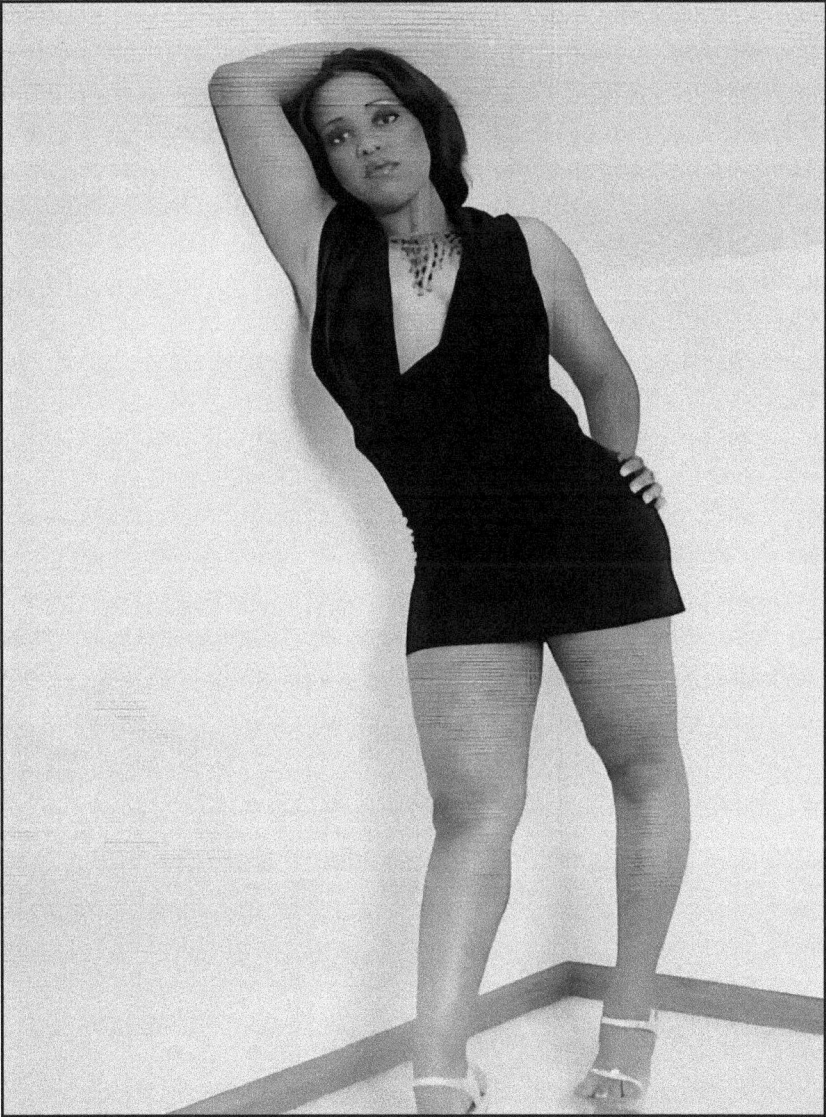

"Relationships"

"You should have been my presence where I go to heal. I have had no peace in this relationship. I have had no rest, only awakened moments of stress. There are no quiet moments, but only echoes of screams and yelling day and night that fall upon my ears. Only rotten words that protrude from your mouth. Only spoken words of agony and pain. Why are you here? I can do fine all by myself. Go away, you shadow of death following me with your darkness. Love doesn't live here anymore. Your loving touch was only a moment in time. Now your touch gives me the chills of a stranger raping me of my dignity. I used to think that I was somebody, but you have made me feel that I am nobody. How could I have ever let you put me in that position of me forgetting me. A position where I have lost my sense of identity. I just wanted you to love me like a calm river that flows gently into the stream, but instead, you loved me like a waterfall that crashes upon the sharp rocks. You leave me with bruises in my heart. Coloring my whole body blue. I thought you would be different than all the rest of my relationships that beat me down and left me wounded like a baby sparrow that has fallen from the sky, struggling to get back up to fly away and spread its wings and try again. You said you were mine until the end of time."

Mena's cousin, Nota, told her, "Mena, get over him. He's nothing but a crutch in your life. I can see right through him, because I am not blinded by love. What has he done for you but taken away the cherished moments in your life? For Real."

Mena thought for a moment about Nota's statement, not being blinded by love.

She even meditated on that thought, and her conclusion was "Men are just like some doctors, they don't believe my pain because some don't see it."

Chapter 13

Hands up (Spider Lily)

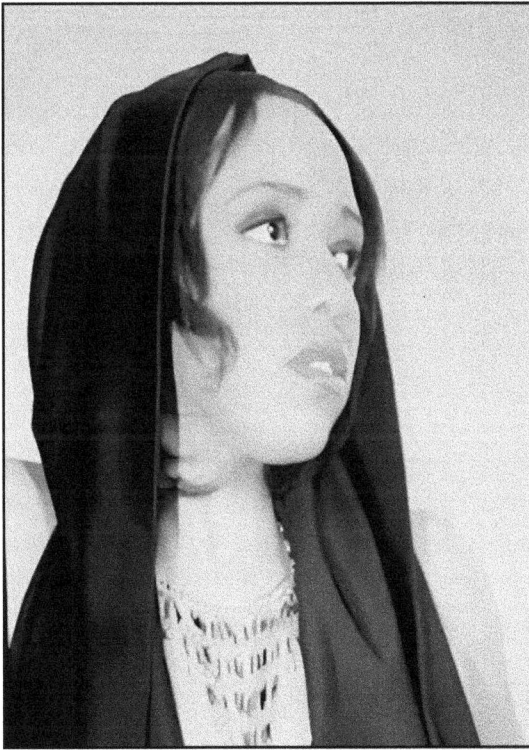

The red spider lily is synonymous with abandonment, loss, death, and separation. But where did this symbolism come from?

They are absolutely gorgeous in the early Autumn, and the vast fields that you see around the Buddhist holiday known as Ohigan and the Autumn Equinox are yet another clear link to the symbolism of this flower. The fact that these flowers bloom only in the Autumn is not the only odd thing about these death flowers. Before the leaves grow, the flower will bloom, and you will see fields of striking red clusters of these long, spidery flowers. They bloom atop long, slender stems, which is why, when they bloom in fields, you will see a gorgeous red carpet of these flowers which can look both beautiful and ethereal. The beauty of these flowers does not last, and they quickly go brown and die, leaving the plant without its browning glory. At this point, the leaves will start to grow, and the plant will start to look alive again before the leaves also turn brown and die, just like the flowers. The fact that these flowers have such a short life span and grow somewhat curiously in comparison to other flowers has baffled people even today. You see, the whole red spider lily is poisonous. The leaves, flowers, and bulbs could kill you in the right doses. **The Red Spider Lily And Why Its Name Is Synonymous With Death-defendersblog https:/defendersblog.org**

Mena read an article in Defenders Blog about these beautiful red spider lily flowers, "The Death Flower Also Known As The Red Spider Lily." It was a Chinese Myth; it was said that the Sun Goddess named Amaterasu, gave two elves the job of guarding the leaves and flowers independently. The guards, Manju and Saka, guarded the petals and the leaves, respectively. Both guards were aware of each other, but they were forbidden to ever meet. But as with any good story, curiosity got the better of them, and they defied the Sun Goddess. The Elvish guards met each other and fell in love. But Amaterasu was not happy with them and decided that they needed to be punished. So, she cursed them to never meet again. This is why Saka's leaves will only grow after Manju's petals have died. They were cursed to live their lives over and over again, eternally separated.

The red Spider lily is often linked with sadness. Mena felt as if she were this Red Spider Lily. She felt as if any relationships that she had had ended in goodbyes, abandonment, awful memories, loss, or death. Why couldn't she be a White Spider Lily, which represented a positive nature, freshness, and simply living life? Why couldn't she be a Golden Lily or a Yellow Spider Lily, which are associated with health and wealth?

Mena thought about a picture that she had taken. Mena thought about the tent of red glowing on her face. She thought about how beautiful she was, yet she was also poisonous. She wore a black cape over her head as if she were mourning for a lost soul. Her beautiful black hair flowing just inches beyond the cape made her look sexy. Enough for a man to gently brush his fingertips upon her hair and face. She remembered how she looked like the Queen of Sheba, with a beaded Black and silver necklace hanging from her long neck, which lingered down to her open breast. It flattered all the guys. Her puckered red lips showed her white teeth ever so slightly. Just enough to arouse and tease a man to want her with desire. She could make a man rejoice in their love together or make his heart die with madness. There were times when she knew that she could make a man drop to his knees, and then there were times when she looked as if death was knocking at her door. The radiance and beauty in her face would turn gray. She would appear as if riding on a pale horse, depicting famine. Just like the Spider Lily, when the flowers turn brown. Looking as if the life within her was being knocked right out of her one day at a time. Then she would perk back up. It would seem as if she were coming back to life just like the leaves on the Spider Lily, but once again, depression would set in, and she was right back on her deathbed.

Mena's First Love

Mena remembered her first love in high school. It was love at first sight. She felt as though she was a gift to him. She thought that she was his pride and joy until one day he hit her. He had a violent temper, and they physically fought often. To ease her pain, Mena began to dabble in marijuana. It made her escape the reality that he wasn't a bad guy. It made her feel like he was always by her side, showing her the way. She had lost all sight of herself. She often missed school just to be with him. Keith dropped out of school in the tenth grade. Mena was now a Senior. Her mother and father often disagreed with many of the things Mena was doing. Especially with the friends she was hanging around with. One day, Mena was missing, and the policeman brought her home. Bruce and Lisa told the police they could keep her. She refuses to abide by our beliefs and the rules of our home.

Earlier that evening, Bruce and Lisa tried to get Mena into the car to go home. Bruce was pulling and pushing Mena to get her in the car. Finally, he gave up and left her there in what they called a rough neighborhood on the other side of town. They had given up. Now, to their surprise, here was the police officer bringing their daughter back to them, saying, 'Until she turns eighteen, you are responsible for her.'

Lisa replied, "Well, I guess you will have to keep bringing her back because she can't stay here, not following the rules of our house. We have to think of the other children's safety."

Lisa would find herself locking her bedroom door at night, afraid of who Mena would bring into the house. Mena finally moved to Baltimore because she no longer felt wanted and had refused to follow the house's rules. Life for her was hard; she felt abandoned. Lisa and Bruce were so heartbroken that they loved Mena so much. Mena's leaving was as if they had been stabbed in their heart with a knife. Keith and Mena had separated, and she hated even looking at his face. One day, she found out in the news that he had to put his "Hands Up." He could no longer live amongst the free society for a while. Keith would be out of her and her son's life for years to come. They never could prove that he was guilty.

Love Life in Baltimore

During Mena's life in Baltimore, there were times when she had to sleep in her car because she had nowhere else to go. She became a professional dancer, which caused her bones to ache with pain. She had to make a living somehow. Mena knew strenuous dancing would cause her to go into a crisis from time to time; however, she couldn't think about it. She had to pay the consequences. It was survival of the fittest. She had to be able to make a living and support herself.

When she was able, Mena would send money home for her son, Mario. He was always in her heart.

She finds her next love, Brutus, an enforcement officer, during one of her performances. What did that name Brutus mean anyway? Mena thought to herself, "I'm going to look it up. Wow! The Deseret News Merriam Webster's editor stated, From the time Shakespeare wrote

Julius Caesar, at the beginning of the 17th century, the name Brutus has been associated with treachery, if not cruelty. The earliest sense of English brutality, which appeared in the 15th century, was typical of a beast. This meaning was derived from a later Latin sense of "Brutus," which had acquired further extended meanings beyond "stupid," such as "irrational" about animals and "thoughtless, inconsiderate" about people." Brutus fits the picture of it all.

Mena thought to herself once again, "He was stupid for leaving the comforts of my arms. He acted like a wild beast, as if he were in control of my thoughts and feelings, going about like a cowardly lion."

Brutus had become irrational when it came to making decisions about Mena's life or his own. He had fallen deep into drugs, finding no way out. He had become thoughtless and irrational in all his ways. Mena would have given him a life of stability. Love should have brought him back into her arms so many times, but he stayed astray, leaving Mena home all alone.

Mena said to herself, "I would have put my 'Hands Up' for him just to be with him. Arrest me. Maybe I'll find him there."

Mena finally walked out of his life, never to return. She didn't know if he was dead or alive to this day.

There were many more that Mena would share her attraction with. She would show her beauty and romance them, dance for them, love them, and finally poison them and break their aching hearts. Then, there were times that they would walk out on her because they couldn't deal with the Sickle Cell crisis that Mena was going through. This was way too much responsibility, something with which they just couldn't deal. It was way too complicated for them.

Wanting to Be Loved

Through all the abuse in life with men. Mena thought about the love of her life, Liam. Her high school sweetheart. His British name means strong-willed warrior. She had always dreamt of the protection he would give her, wrapped up in his arms, only to find out that they were cousins. He always protected her and their friendship, both during her high school years and as they matured into adults. One of her best friends had stolen his heart away. She had heard through the grapevine that Liam had died a sudden death. Mena hadn't even bothered to pick up the phone to call. Mena didn't offer her condolences because they hadn't been on speaking terms in a long while. Even though she wanted to so badly, Mena decided to leave their broken friendship in the past. Mena thought about the days when they used to talk, and one of the things they would discuss was Sherry's name. Sherry's name means "darling" and "beloved." Mena and Liam would laugh and giggle about how old Sherry's name was. Mena would always tease Sherry and say, "Come here, darling." Sherry was deeply loved by her husband, Liam. Mena had wondered if they had stayed together and weren't cousins, would he have loved her as much as he had loved Sherry? That's a memory that Mena always kept buried in the back of her mind.

Time to Try Again

Mena had decided, after her failed marriage, that she would never marry again. When Mena and her family returned home to live, she came across an old schoolmate whom she used to know. His name was Adam. Mena felt it was time to try again with a new relationship. They were a wonderful team. They fished together, coached basketball together, partied together, had cookouts together, drank together, and got high together. The drinking and getting high were a bit too much. Could this have become the downfall of their relationship? Mena didn't think so, she felt that the medical marijuana known as medical cannabis truly alleviates symptoms and treats medical conditions. Even more so was the strain of his presence in her home with her oldest kids. Mario and Amelia had had enough of men whom they thought were no good for their mother. Rex made things even worse by telling lies to Bree and Boxer about Adam. Mena thought that his name fitted him perfectly. Adam's name means being fruitful and multiplying on the earth. Adam was in so much debt due to having many children. He was being fruitful and multiplying on the earth with his eight kids. Mena knew that she would never bear him any children; the four she had already had really taken a toll on her body. Adam's name also meant created from the earth. Adam was an earthly person. He never looked groomed, and he always smelled of the earth. What she liked about him most of all was that he was a down-to-earth person. He loved nature and kids. He tried his best to cater to Mena's children, but it just wasn't in the cards for him to do so. Mena and Adam argued frequently about the smallest and simplest things, especially regarding the children. So, Adam has just given up on trying to discipline them and instead caters to them. He felt that his best was never good enough. Mena had put him out of the house twice. The reason for doing so was that she felt that if he couldn't be there for her in the hospital and support her through her most challenging times of struggling to stay alive, then she just didn't need him. His defense was that he just couldn't stand the sight of being in the hospital. Even when he did visit, all they did was argue. Even when Adam would call, they would argue. Mena was always about what he should have or could have been doing for her and her family. He felt that he was doing more for Mena's family than his own.

Get To Steppin

Once again, Mena would become upset and direct her anger in the wrong direction at anyone she came into contact with. Mena felt as though she were breaking down once again from another relationship. Sure enough, the relationship was off, but they remained friends. During the arguments that they would have, it would cause her stress, and of course, her crisis got worse. Mena felt like something was crawling and invading her body, which caused her to have muscle spasms. She felt like her body was once again going down to the ground. She was burning with agony from the inside to the outside. Burns would appear on her face. She knew that in Africa, Sickle Cell would fight off Malaria, but what was causing the burns on her body and face? For what was her body fighting? Could it be OxyContin, which is a time-release version of oxycodone.) Not to mention the Dilaudid pills of 2 milligrams that took up to 3 hours to work some of her pain away. Mena was sure that there was way too much medicine in her system at the time. At times, she experienced the common side effects: constipation, nausea or vomiting, stomach discomfort, feelings of sleepiness or tiredness, dizziness and vertigo, itchiness or rash, headaches, and confusion. There were times when Mena couldn't even lift her head. Adam and Mena argued a lot because Mena would think that she had told him something or had forgotten what she might have said to him. That was the way it was for many who would try to have a conversation with Mena when she was on OxyContin and Oxycodone. Through it all, there was always someone there supporting her and helping to take care of the children. Of course, Mario and Amelia were much older now, so they helped to make sure that Bree and Boxer stayed on schedule and were well taken care of, not to mention Mum Mum, Pup Pup, her brother and sisters, uncles, aunts, cousins, and her friends. There were times when Fentanyl and Morphine were given as well. Mena would sometimes just find herself as an object of just existing. Adam just couldn't deal with it all. So, he went steppin' as Mena requested him to. She threw her "Hands Up" at him as well.

Chapter 14

Rare Sighting (Two Moons)

Rare Sighting—An occasion when you see something or someone, especially something that is rare or trying to hide. Sighting/definition in the Cambridge English Dictionary. http://dictionary. cambridge.org. A sight that is not common and isn't to be seen regularly. The rarest sighting would be two moons. It has only been seen once in Japan. "Urban Dictionary" https://www.urbandictionary.com (Al Overview). It's usually an optical illusion caused by atmospheric conditions like temperature inversions, or rare cases, could be a temporary "mini-moon" —a small asteroid captured by Earth's gravity for a short period, which would be too faint to see with the naked eye. Earth has one natural moon.

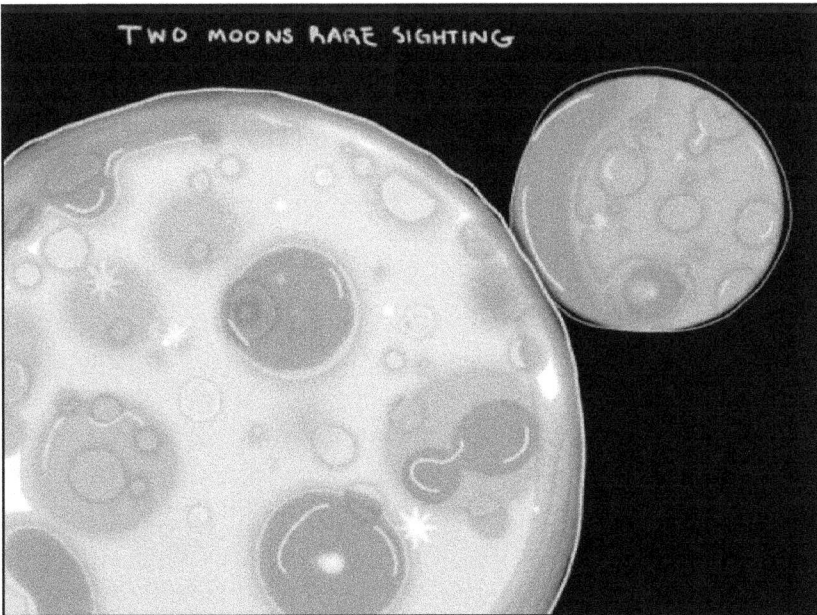

TWO MOONS RARE SIGHTING

One day, Mena's mom was swimming, and the water was a deep, rich, dark blue color with the rarest formation of clouds; a beautiful sight caught Lisa's eye. It was an incredibly special moment that she didn't often see. It was an occasion that filled her heart with joy. It was like the rare sighting of two moons, something you don't see regularly. Lisa had spotted Mena among the bright green clumps of tall, green-bladed grass with dark blue skylight water under the elegant sky. The best way Lisa could encapsulate this moment was to compare Mena to what many Caucasians would conceive of as beautiful: a blonde, white woman with long, flowing hair blowing in the wind and glistening in the sun. What Lisa saw that day was the image of her daughter glowing like Queen Nzinga Mbande of Ndongo, a feminist ancestor. Her name means 'proud daughter of the soil' —an Afrikaner, which refers to whites living in South Africa. The name was symbolic in many ways and would later prove to be a harbinger of a tumultuous, charismatic, and eventful life. These characteristics are fitting for a queen, among the greatest rulers of the Alkebulan people. She was a woman, a Black hero, a fierce warrior whose struggle against white imperialism in Africa is recorded as one of the greatest in history. Arts & Culture "Afro Lady" afrolady. com. Mena's hair was not blowing in the wind at all. Mena's hair was pulled up in a bun with curls, with no special order. It was a natural crown placed upon her head. Lisa humbly bowed her head to see such a sight as the waves were ripping up and down. Mena was smiling, relaxed, and elated with joy. Lisa was noticing something in her daughter that was often missing. Lisa's heart skipped a beat to see this glimpse of her daughter, a picture of Art.

Lisa spoke aloud, unable to contain herself, and said, "A Kodak moment."

Mena's life had been nothing but tumultuous, charismatic, and eventful—a story meant to be told. Mena wants to be a legendary warrior who the books of history will never forget. Just as Nzinga helped uplift education and innovation among her people. Mena wanted to educate and inform the public about Sickle Cell. She would seek to improve science and technology to conquer this incurable disease. She would be charismatic. She was going to attract, influence, and inspire as many people as possible with her personal qualities, because sometimes her characteristics would turn others away, and nobody would be listening. One day, she was bound to be noticed by people everywhere throughout the world.

Lisa could not even begin to describe the sky that day. It was just a rare sight to see. It looked like snow in the sky with the sun taking its last breath of the day, fighting to shine ever so brightly. The sky reminded Lisa of the cream custard her mother, Ann, used to make. The sky was so appetizing that it looked good enough to eat. Sometimes you couldn't tell where the sky began or ended. It was like seeing two moons, a reflection in her eyes. It truly was an afternoon delight. Mena was so refined and poised, helping her son to learn how to fish. Lisa could not hear a single thing that they were saying, but she knew Mena was spending a rare moment of bonding and being the mom she always wanted to be. Mena was able to enjoy her every waking moment without pain. She had pushed aside the swollen hands that would later sneak up on her and bring her into the beginning of excruciating pain Sickle Cell crisis. It was truly a rare moment, and Lisa was able to participate in it from a distance. Oh, and her smile was joined instantly by her son. Mena took a picture of that rare moment. They were happy, at least in that moment. A scene that was often taken for granted by many, but Lisa knew better.

Chapter 15

Mena's Waking Moments and Sleepless Nights (Different Phases of The Moon)

Moon—The eight lunar phases are, in order: new moon, waxing crescent, first quarter, waxing gibbous, full moon, waning gibbous, third quarter, and waning crescent. The cycle repeats once a month (every 29.5 days).

https://science.nasa.gov New: We cannot see the Moon when it is a New Moon. Waxing Crescent: In the Northern Hemisphere, we see the waxing crescent phase as a thin crescent of light on the right. First Quarter: We see the first quarter phase as a half-moon. Waxing Gibbous: The waxing gibbous phase is between a half-moon and a full moon. https://www.kopernik.org

Lisa described Mena's waking and sleeping hours as the sight of the moon. One phase would be a Waning Gibbous Moon. During this phase, Mena could be seen in the early morning daylight hours. Moving ever so slowly. Mena was experiencing fatigue; however, she knew that she had to balance her inner needs. She had a pull within her for solitude and introspection. She felt lonely and unwanted. She had to balance her external responsibilities to her family. She knew that she had plenty of duties as a mother, such as household chores, taking care of the bills, scheduling doctor's appointments, and scheduling teachers' appointments. She would wake up with a mix of emotions, but she knew it was time for her to shine, so the kids could see that she was genuinely interested in their education. She felt that meditating in bed would serve her best; however, this was not the time for self-reflection. It was something she loved to do when she was alone, thinking about releasing some of her old habits and considering how she could transform the unwanted situation she was in into something positive. The kids loved the special attention they received from their mom, filled with hugs and kisses. Through it all, Mena loved the feeling of being up, making sure the kids were off and ready for school. She loved watching the kids as they ran down the long driveway, waving goodbye. Boxer would always be first, and he would never tire out because, through his boxing training, he was always first in the crowd of boys and girls who had to run at least a mile for warm-up. His mother would be late arriving for practice most of the time, so when they arrived there, he would place his things in the locker room and then run as fast as he could to catch up with the group and speed past them. That was the only benefit of his mother running late. It kept him in good shape. Bree, on the other hand, would quickly run out of breath, but she never gave up and would make the bus. Not only that, but it also seemed to affect her side, which was causing her pain for some unknown reason. This was something that Bree had complained about for quite some time. If only Mena could stay well enough to finish addressing the problem with all the testing and places the doctors were sending them before another crisis would bring Mena down once again into the dark room, Mena would go through a phase where her waking hours would be between 9 pm and Midnight. Mena's illuminations on her face seemed to get less and less of a glow as the days went on. This illumination is constantly changing and can vary. That was the way Mena was. You just had to take it one day at a time. She would rise later and later each night, setting after sunrise in the morning. This is the first phase after the Full Moon.

You can't see the New Moon because it is next to the sun; it's much brighter than anything else in the sky. Another reason you can't see it is that it is positioned between us and the Sun. That's the way the kids felt about their mother. The closed door to Mena's bedroom would put a division between her and the kids. That off-white door would serve as a barrier to hiding the illuminating light and the presence of their mother's face. They knew that the room was dark and gloomy, keeping her away from them. They couldn't wait for this phase to pass because the laughter and joy of the family were gone during these times of darkness. There was loneliness that filled the air. The house felt cold with no warmth. There were no fuzzy kisses from their mother. There were no rules. The schedule placed on the refrigerator meant nothing to them. The bright-lit side of the Moon is facing away from us. Only the dark, unlit side is facing toward us. Mena was experiencing a lack of energy during this time. The New Moon mostly made Mena vulnerable to thinking about times when she was hurting emotionally within her hidden cells. It left her unmotivated and extremely tired. So, how does the moon become visible to us? Every day, the moon rises around 50 minutes later than it did the day before. A few days after the New Moon, it rises a few hours after the Sun and is almost impossible to see in the bright sky. Mena emerges from the closed door to use the bathroom. But as the Sun sets, a slender crescent appears. The children catch a glimpse of their mother as she takes a peek around the house and returns to her room. It's as if a cloud passed over that part of the moon for a breath moment. Mena missed her kids so much that's why she would make an appearance, wishing she could be more present for them. She knew that the meds that kept her down in silence and the pain that caused her to struggle to walk were affecting her kids. She had to take action to be there for them. She had to overcome every obstacle to be the mother they wanted her to be.

Overall, half of the Moon (Waxing Crescent) is always in sunlight, and half in darkness. As the Moon orbits Earth, it changes just how much of the lit side we can see. A few days later, it rises around midday and is visible in the blue afternoon sky.

The children's faces begin to light up as Mena finally wakes up at noon to ask, "Did you guys eat? Did you feed the birds? Did you do your chores? What day is it?"

As seen from Earth, the Moon is 90 degrees from the Sun, and exactly half its face is illuminated. This is the First Quarter Moon because the Moon has gone one-quarter of the way around the Earth. Remember, it rises about two weeks after the New Moon, minutes later than the day before, at sunset.

The full Moon is the only phase where the Moon is up for the whole night. Every now and then, Mena would feel refreshed. Mena felt as though the Full Moon gave her a feeling of starting anew. It motivated her to get things done. Lisa and the children knew that Mena would be up all night. Illuminating with smiles and singing. She would have come to life watching movies all night long with them. They would have popcorn, ice cream, and Chinese food throughout the night. Their mom was back. The crisis had succeeded. The Moon is now on the opposite side of the Earth from the Sun, and the side facing us is completely illuminated. Their mom was back; she had filled the house with dance and laughter again. They would have double rays of light. The moonlight and the sunshine. This is the halfway point of the lunar month. And the Moon continues to rise later and later—about a week after the Full Moon.

The Third Quarter Moon rises around midnight. As before, half of the Moon's face is illuminated. But it's the other way round to the First Quarter Moon two weeks ago. A few days after Half Moon, it shrinks away again, rising as a thin crescent (Waning Crescent) just before sunrise, and once more, it's lost in the glare of the Sun. As the Moon passes between the Earth and the Sun, we're back at the New Moon again. Lisa knew that was exactly the way Mena was; it could happen in the opposite direction. It's been just over four weeks since the last New Moon. And the lunar cycle begins again. Sometimes that lunar crisis cycle of Mena's would begin too soon.

What was the kid's favorite Moon Phase?

Lisa spoke to herself in her mind. "It definitely would be the Bright Full Moon."

That is the one Lisa would have chosen as well, along with Mena's entire family and friends. Which one would be Mena's choice: a delicate crescent Moon, A bright Full Moon, or a Quarter Moon against the blue sky? Mena, by choice, loved them all.

Chapter 16

The Next Visit (Salmon & Fiddler Crabs)

Salmon use a combination of olfaction(smell) and sensing of the Earth's magnetic field to find their way home. Fiddler crabs count their steps and track the distance of each step to calculate how far they've traveled from home. A process known as path integration. https://iobopen.com

Birds do it, bees do it, and so do rats, and cats. It is homing: finding your way back home even after traveling long distances over unfamiliar territory.

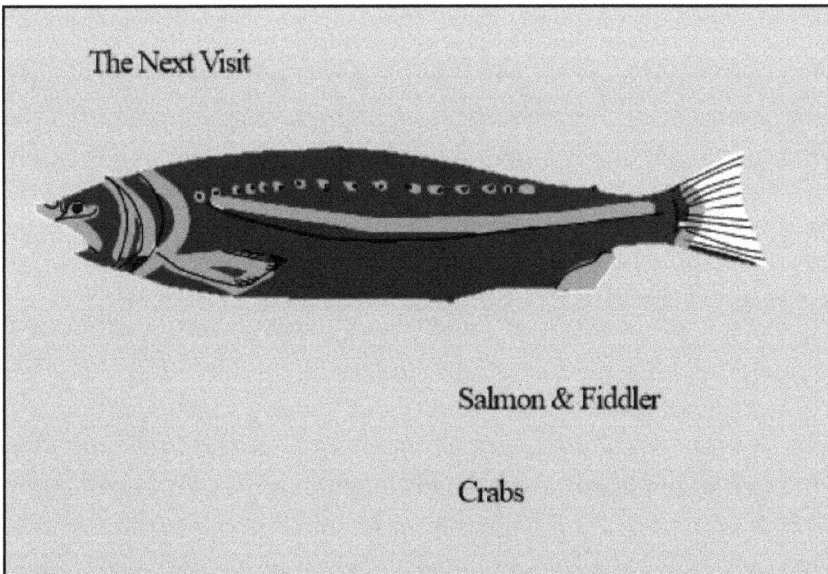

The Next Visit

Salmon & Fiddler

Crabs

Loss of Mena's Uncle

This time, the visit was not to the home hospital. Lisa had to travel to a hospital that was three hours away to be with Mena. Mena was undergoing a special procedure. It dealt with having a port placed in her chest. Mena had a device implanted in her chest so that they could draw blood, administer medications, or fluids. Mena's veins had been stuck so many times because they could not get access to the bloodstream without repeatedly sticking her. Her veins were bruised and unusable. Lisa had developed a fear of driving on the road as she got older. She knew deep in her heart that she had to deal with the memory of losing her brother, Cedrick, whose name means "kindly and loved," and also the gift of splendor. He was always giving her mother gifts that came from the heart, such as handmade pictures, blankets, cups, etc. The picture showed every family member looking out of a window, with her mother and father at the open window of a house. The picture was drawn with black ink. He died in a car wreck. He was killed by a tractor-trailer on a mountaintop. They said that Lisa's brother, Cedrick, had fallen asleep at the wheel on the way home. What a likely story. He was running for governor in the county where he lived. There were a few people who didn't want that to happen, but the majority of the people in the county absolutely loved him.

Lisa's mother, Ann, was never the same after that. She died of a broken heart. It had affected Lisa, making her extremely nervous about tractor-trailers on the road. She could only think of the horrible accident in which her brother didn't survive. Lisa was in her first year of college, and he was only twenty-one when he died. It made Lisa even more nervous when she didn't know where she was going, especially if she had to travel on the Beltway in Maryland.

The Stressful Ride to The Hospital

Oh, how she wished she were a Salmon or a Fiddler Crab, knowing her way to the hospital where her daughter, Mena, seemed to be spending more time. It had come to be like Mena's second home. If Lisa could fly like a bird to her destination in unfamiliar territory, she would. Lisa didn't like plane rides either because she was afraid of heights. Lisa's ears would clog up, and she would feel dizzy. She knew it was her Sickle Cell Trait that was giving her these side effects.

Salmon and Fiddlers sense the Earth's magnetic field. Lisa compared her GPS for that same description. It would tell her how to get to the hospital across the bridge that was 300 miles away, and she knew that it would work the same way to help her find her way back home.

Listening to the Words of The Nurse

Finally, Lisa arrived at the hospital. Lisa walked into Mena's room to ask her more questions, but instead, she sat down listening to the conversation between Mena and the nurse. Lisa looked at the board, and the nurse's name was Lily. What a beautiful name. Lisa's grandmother's name was Lily. It signifies purity and innocence. Lisa was thinking to herself, describing the way the nurse looked at her. She is young with pretty, long auburn hair. She seemed to have a look as if she were from the Dominican Republic. Her long, slender fingers had nails polished in white and gold. They were, of course, short, but well-manicured. Her voice was as gentle as a whisper, so Lisa had to listen very closely to every word she was saying.

Mena said, "Hi, Mom! Lily, this is my mother."

Lily acknowledged her by saying, "Hello, you look as young as your daughter. I would never have pictured you as Mena's mother. I thought you were her sister."

They both took the focus off of Lisa when Mena said, "Are you holding it side to side?"

Lily said, "Hum, I have it top to bottom. Do you want it this way?"

Mena replied, "Not top bottom, it has to be horizontal because you're not going to get it. You got to hold it tight because it will move on you."

Lisa was learning about how a port is accessed. She couldn't hear the next thing the nurse was saying because the TV was extremely loud. It was saying that "If President Obama had declared it to be a disaster area instead of just a state of emergency. The state of emergency only gives us a five-million-dollar cap. If they had submitted it for a Disaster Declaration, we could have gotten ninety-six dollars or more. The president had already denied the request once, stating that the situation with the pledge was man-made. This is CBS News."

Lisa turned her attention back to what was going on with Mena. Lisa thought to herself, "My daughter has gone through this procedure so many times that she is telling the nurse what to do." Lisa thought about this situation again to herself, "How could I not know the pain and the procedures that my daughter has been going through?" Lisa was feeling ashamed and out of touch with her daughter.

There was a pause in the noise of the TV, and Lily asked, "You feel better?"

Mena asked, "Is it returning and flushing, okay? It's sore from."

Lily interrupted, "Uhm, from all the stabs. Multiple stab wounds."

Mena laughed and said, "Are you trying to kill me, women?" Mena and Lily laughed. Mena said, "It's a multipurpose stab wound."

Lily said, "No, I hate stabbing people, all in the same spot too."

Lilly was holding something that resembled a large plastic bandage with a hole in the middle and two handles on the sides. All of a sudden, there was a noise coming from it that sounded like a pig oink, oink, oink, oink.

Lilly said, "This is a different kind of…"

Mena interrupted Lily, saying, "It's a Meng Tegaderm. I don't like it; it's got a white border."

Lily said, "Oh, you don't like this kind?"

Mena answered her and said, "Either way, my skin is going to be irritated."

Lisa could hear the background noise of the loud TV discussing the weather. "Low decrees, it's going to be a big problem for your car. A Milton mechanic tells ABC News station that the most important thing is to keep an eye on your antifreeze. It's a wind chill on the front of your radiator. If you go down the road on a day like today, you have to have enough antifreeze to protect it, to keep it protected, to keep it from freezing."

Then loud music played when the news was going off. Lisa was trying so hard to keep her focus on what was happening that darn TV was distracting her, and it was turned up so loud.

Mena said, "Is that the plastic tape?"

Lilly said, "Uhm, you like that other stuff, don't you?"

Mena responded, "Yell."

Lily said, "Something like sign it, I can properly document that the needle was also due to a change."

Lily had laughed in the middle of her conversation, so Lisa didn't know what Lily was trying to say because the TV was screaming at her. Lily's whole two sentences didn't make any sense to Lisa. Then Mena and Lily both laughed. The procedure had been accomplished. Mena had taught Lily and Lisa how to access a port. Mena had used Lily as the tool to follow her directions. This procedure took three minutes.

Lisa thought, "*Thank goodness that procedure was all over. All that to get blood.*"

Chapter 17

I'M Free (Briar)

Briar—any number of prickly, scrambling shrubs, especially the sweetbrier and other wild roses. The name Briar-Rose is evidently the famous symbol that the beautiful roses are always associated with thorns that defend themselves painfully. Here, of course, we again think of our pure soul as the epitome of beauty and love that awakens and blossoms like a beautiful rose under the spring sun. (https://foilagefriend.com) Any of many plants with thorny stems growing in dense clusters.

Mena combed her hair that morning. She looked as youthful as a princess. She had parted her hair in the middle, creating two ponytails. It made Lisa think of her when she was a little girl. Mena was her little princess. Lisa compared her to a Briar Rose. Mena was quite beautiful today, and yet she had a tube protruding from the side of her neck that felt like a prickly rose thorn. Mena was standing her ground in explaining and defending herself to the Nurse on how to go about getting this tube out of her neck. She was defending herself and explaining how the first nurse, Lily, had assisted her with the dressing she had. The sun was beaming through the window ever so brightly, causing Mena to glow like a bright colored rose. A good night's sleep had done Mena well. She was definitely a blossom of beauty, for she had awakened with a smile on her face, even though she was complaining that her body felt like thorns touching every inch of her skin.

The Nurse Hope, whose name means positive expectation, wanted to know about her patient's Sickle Cell; however, she focused on her job first and asked, "Is this your dressing, Mena?"

Mena replied, "Ah-hon."

Hope said, "You have little fine hairs up there. Oh my gosh. Sorry, does it hurt Mena? Feels like it hurts those little fine hairs."

Mena replied, "My nurse helped me with the last piece in the back, so she probably did that."

Mena let out a small snicker. Mena went on to say proudly, "I could have been a nurse. I still could if my Sickle Cell would calm down."

Explanation of Sickle Cell

Now the opportunity had presented itself for Hope to ask her questions about Sickle Cell, but before Hope could really think about it, she blurted out, "Are they still supposed to be, like still working on a cure for that?"

Mena was prepared as usual to answer any questions that needed answering during her hospital stay. It's time to school another person was all that she was thinking. Finally, Mena said, "Gene Cell Therapy, but it's still…" then Hope interrupted and said, "Uh-huh, whew."

Mena continued on with her conversation, "But they don't want to have a cure." Hope said, "Like cancer?" And then Mena said, "They don't want to cure that either."

"They have a cure for it." Hope vented, "Yeah, I often wonder why you can't, maybe it is because it's because everybody's DNA is different, everybody's different, and all cancers are different, so you can't treat everybody the same because everybody's different."

Hope was working continuously throughout their conversation, getting the tube out of Mena's neck. She said, "Let me turn the tube to one side, all right?"

Mena replied. "Yeah, but you've got to start from somewhere."

Mena looked up at Hope with frustration in her eyes that a cure hadn't been found for all too quick enough. Mena pursed her lips and sighed.

Hope continued to ask more questions while she continued to try to withdraw the tube from Mena's neck slowly, but surely. "Yeah,

I often wonder, like you know, Sickle Cell, is it normally in African Americans?"

Hope began to talk to herself again while trying to remove the tube. The tube looked disgusting. It was a white tube protruding out of the left side of Mena's neck, like a worm coming out of an apple, except the area around it was bloody and rotten-looking. Mena's bruise was the color of burgundy.

Hope went on with her questions, "When you have people who are mixed, when you have, like you know, a Caucasian and African American can have offspring who are mixed, can they have Sickle Cell?"

Mena's words came rolling out of her mouth, dying to answer those questions. These were questions that she had answered all her life. Mena was described as mixed. Her father was of mixed Black and white descent from the Mediterranean area, and her mother was African American, with genes from Blackstone, Virginia, and Indian ancestry.

Mena answered, "Yeah, they can!"

Hope was relieved, "I've often wondered that."

Mena, "Well..." Pausing way too long to speak.

Hope went on to say, "Have they studied even that?"

Mena quickly answered this time, "Well, the thing is, I've got parents who have Sickle Cell trait."

Hope was bewildered, "Huh. Oh, Oh gosh. So, it can come from down the line?"

Mena said, "Oh, yell cause like even some Mediterranean, like some of those they carry it."

Mena nodded her head, "like some of them have Hemoglobin C. So, what it is, is somebody dipped somewhere."

They both begin to laugh hysterically out loud in amusement. Mena went on to say, "They were doing a lot of dipping back in the day."

Hope said, "Okay, gotcha, all right, hey Mena, they were dippin and switchin."

Hope was Caucasian, and she mentioned, "I had somebody in my past, he was African American, and he was a cutie."

Mena explained, "That's how uh Sickle Cell has come to be in different races like in the Caribbean."

Mena thought about a time when she was a teenager and a white girl asked her if she washes her hair. She thought about how she could ask her such a question. Were white people that obvious, wondering how we clean ourselves? She was feeling the same way about this nurse, not knowing much about Sickle Cell, and yet she was in the hands of Hope, taking care of her. Throughout all the laughter and conversation between Mena and Hope, Mena was left with a bad feeling in her insides. She was feeling as if she had a thorn in her side.

Removal of the Tube

Finally, the moment had arrived. Hope said, "Mena, take a deep breath and breathe out."

Hope removed the tube very gently from Mena's neck as Mena did as told. Mena could finally breathe through her mouth and nose. Mena's voice sounded different and weak. Yet she managed to say, "I'm free! It feels like a huge briar has been taken out of my neck. I am free from the restraints of this tube that was implanted in my neck. I now have the power to advocate freely without the soreness in my throat to speak."

Mena had once again navigated an uncomfortable situation without breaking down. She had courage and knowledge about the port because she had been through this procedure before. Being able to share what she knew with Hope took a lot of the focus off of what her body was going through.

Lisa was overwhelmed with tears at the sight of her daughters smiling so brightly, and her laugh was so genuine. She had realized the strength Mena had in controlling what was taking place with her body. It was like watching a rose finally open after a long winter.

Chapter 18

Rainy Days and Mondays
Always Get Me Down
(Rhododendrons)

Rhododendrons are definitely eye-catching, for they have large clusters of spring blooms. They grew 4/to 15' tall and wide. Rhododendrons contain poisonous substances and should not be ingested by humans or animals. Honey made from flowers may also be toxic. All parts of this flower are poisonous, highly toxic, and may be fatal if eaten. Rhododendron grows into huge bushes with thick vegetation that blocks out sunlight and smothers most other wild plants and trees, stopping them from growing or regenerating. https://www.gardenia.net.

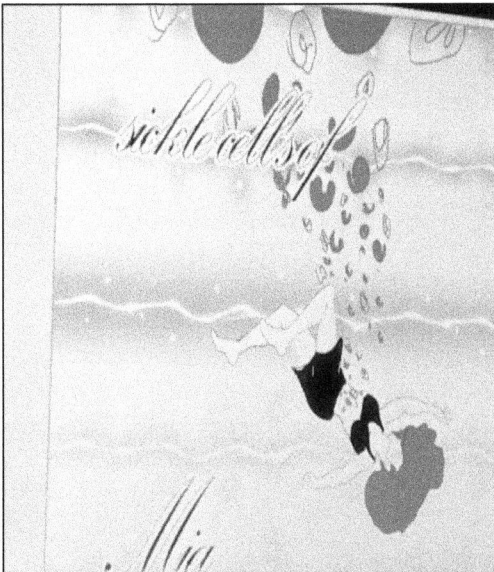

Mena thought to herself on Monday morning that the State of Washington was beautiful. It was full of rhododendrons. Mena said to herself, "Why would such a beautiful flower want to grow in such a rainy place?"

The rain didn't help with Mena's depression. She didn't feel like getting up out of bed, washing up, doing household chores, cooking, or seeing anyone. Not even her children. She could hear the house waking up. The dog, Skipper, was running back and forth as if he were the captain of a ship at the sound of Boxer's footsteps. Skipper thought he was the boss of the household.

Mena thought, "Why couldn't Boxer, for once, walk like a normal person?"

Boxer, just like Skipper, was running around quickly about the house. Bree had uncovered the birds, and they were chirping as loud as they possibly could, waiting to be fed and welcoming the morning sun. Mena didn't mind that too much because the birds always brought music to their ears. They helped Mena start her engine in her brain to have a great mental start, and today they were helping her brain relax. Soon, she would hear the sound of Amelia in the bathroom doing her daily routine. Next would come the yelling and screaming of everyone wanting to use the master bathroom.

Bree would be the first. "Amelia, I have to go to the bathroom." Boxer was already in the other bathroom. Bree yelled, "Can you both hurry up?"

Amelia screamed, "If you wanted to use the bathroom, you should have gotten up earlier."

Bree screamed back, "When do you suggest dawn?"

She had heard that saying in the movie A Raisin in the Sun.

Next came the pounding of the door. Bree said, "Hurry up, I have to go; I'm going to pee on myself."

Boxer finally came out, and Bree would go running down the hallway to the other bathroom, knocking Boxer to the ground without saying "excuse me."

Then, the crying began, and the knocking on the door started. "Mommie, Bree knocked me down without saying excuse me. Mommie! Mommie!"

Mena could hear Mario adding to the morning noise, shouting, "Quit knocking on the door. You know that mom didn't get any sleep last night, and she's going to start yelling at you both."

Amelia finally came out the door and said, "Shut up, Boxer, mom's going to come out and start

yelling at everyone. Next, you know she's going to start telling everyone what to do, especially you, because you didn't do the dishes last night."

"Bree, tell Boxer you're sorry."

Mario banged on the door Bree was in because he now had to use the bathroom. The next thing you know, he had punched a hole in the door. He didn't even really care because in his mind, he knew all that his mother was going to do was yell at him, and that would be the end of it. Someone would fix it.

The Pain Settling In

Mena couldn't even address the situation because just like that, overnight, her body had gone into another crisis. Her shoulder and her side were keeping her tied down to her bed. This was going to be a bad one.

Mena thought to herself, "It may not be just a Blood Transfusion, but a Blood Exchange." She would have to worry about all the going on in her house at another time. Not today, but maybe tomorrow.

Mena felt as if she were in another place and time. She felt as if her body was being taken over by something strange. Her body felt as if a rhododendron was taking it over and smothering out all the good cells in her body. She felt as if her body, soul, and mind were in a dark place.

Back At The Hospital

There was no sunshine in her life. There was no family, friends, or lover accompanying her right now at this moment at the hospital. Her mental capacity was being poisoned inch by inch. She was in a toxic environment. Doctors, nurses, dietary aids, and environmentalists once again surrounded her. The hospital was one of the least clean places you could possibly want to be. Mena pushed the button.

The nurse came in. "How can I help you, Mena?"

Mena looked at the whiteboard that was on the wall and asked, "Are you the charge nurse, April?" Mena thought in her mind that April means moving forward in a new and positive way. April was supposed to be about beauty, growth, and youth. Currently, there was nothing in her life that was new or moving in a positive direction. There was no beauty in her or the nurse that she could see. All Mena could see was the growth of Sickled Cells growing throughout her entire body, taking over her whole cells. Her body was dying as if winter was creeping in on it. Life was moving slowly. She was entering another period, Death.

Handle This Please

Mena went on to say, "My sheets are dirty, the floor is dirty, and the bathroom is disgusting. How can anyone get well in this filthy environment?" Mena mustered up all the energy that was left in her and threw the sheets on the floor, yelling and screaming. "I need someone to please handle this situation now. I can't possibly lie in this bed. Let alone walk on these floors."

Mena collapsed in the chair beside the bed with her IV attached to her in misery.

The nurse, April, replied, "I will get someone right away to take care of this situation."

Mena had been to the hospital so many times that all the nurses now knew who she was. When Mena arrived, only the charge nurse was allowed to care for Mena. They all knew Mena knew her rights as a patient and that she was an advocate for other patients who entered the hospital with Sickle Cell. The situation was managed right away, and believe me, Mena directed the environmentalist on every aspect of what she wanted cleaned. The environmentalist could feel Mena's peering eyes upon her with every step she made.

Mena would say, "Can you get that spot? It looks like mold is growing in that corner. Please don't use that dirty rag on the sink; you just used it for the toilet, that's nasty. The chairs in here need cleaning for when visitors come. I know it won't be many, but still, it doesn't matter how many visitors come, that's the point of it all."

The environmentalist mumbled under her breath, "I see why she doesn't get many visitors."

Mena would just go on and on with her list of things for the environmentalist to do. Finally, the job was done, and the environmentalist left as quickly as possible before another thought could enter Mena's head. Mena climbed back into bed, looking all around to make sure there wasn't a spot of dirtiness on the sheets. She moved the sheets back and forth, back and forth, before she proceeded to crawl into bed.

When she was satisfied, she left an awkward note for the nurse, which said, "October 6, April (RN). It'll make me feel safe if you page my doctor, so I can get the best possible care. They know me, they know me best."

No Peace of Mind

Mena fell fast asleep from exhaustion to find peace of mind. She knew that when she would awaken, she would return right back to another time and place in her life where she didn't want to be.

Sure enough, she was awakened by the sound of the doctor's voice saying, "Mena, I have your report on your blood results."

There was no warm greeting, such as 'hello,' 'good afternoon,' or 'how are you feeling?' Was she just another number in his desire to make the day end? Did he have any feelings or interest in Mena being a human being at all? Was she more knowledgeable about Sickle Cell than he was? Did he even know what the numbers meant? Doctors read off the numbers WBC 4.0, MCV 80, MCH 28.1, MCHC 35.3, RDW 21.8, PLT 69, MPV 8.8, RBC 2.92, Hemo 8.2, Hematocrit 23.3.

The doctor said, "We will continue to give you Dilaudid, Benadryl, and Oxycodone. Your body is making more Sickle Cells than whole cells. We are going to have to give you a blood exchange instead of a transfusion."

Mena's mind was prepared for this, but not her heart. She called her mother to tell her about it, and all her mom could say was, "Mena, you know I can't stand the sight of blood. I can't watch the bag of blood hanging in your room."

Mena replied, "I have to go downstairs to get the blood exchange, so you wouldn't see a bag hanging. That's a blood transfusion. You don't have to come, I'm used to being by myself."

Not knowing the severity of it, Lisa said, "I will come and visit you a little later on."

Mena replied, "You don't have to, I'm fine."

Lisa said, "I want to."

Confrontation

Lisa hadn't visited Mena very often because Mena slept on and off a lot, and Mena seemed as if she were Bipolar. There were times when the visit was quite pleasant and times when it wasn't pleasant at all. Mena argued with the Doctors, Nurses, Dietitians, and just about anyone who came into the room. It seemed as if Mena and Lisa disagreed about everything all the time. Lisa felt as if she was walking on shells, trying to make sure that she was saying the right thing. They both agreed that being together wasn't the best thing, and yet they loved each other very much. Lisa felt incredibly happy inside when her daughter would call her for advice or ask her to help solve a problem. Lisa felt that her daughter still needed her, but it was strange that they never seemed to agree on anything. It was two mothers butting heads.

Mena asked her mom, "Can you ask the nurse to bring me a knife?" Lisa replied, "I don't think now is the time; a man is screaming next door who needs the nurse's attention."

Mena would say, "I'm sure not all of them are attending to him."

Lisa said, "Okay, I will go and see if I can find one."

Lisa walked out the door, and there was no one in sight. Lisa came back in and said, "I didn't see anyone. They are attending to the man who is screaming."

Mena pressed the button, and a nurse came along. Mena said, "Can you bring me a knife?"

The nurse said, "Sure, I'll get you one."

Lisa said, "Why did you do that? They were busy. I don't think a knife is important right now."

Mena replied, "They are here to take care of me, that's what their job is."

Lisa muzzled her mouth so that something as simple as this situation wouldn't turn into a huge argument. She knew that she needed to keep Mena's stress level down. She didn't want to make Mena angry or start crying. Her Sickle Cell Crisis caused Mena to become emotionally upset in so many directions. The visits could get or seem extremely complicated. You either left hurt and angry, happy, or joyous. Most of the time, it was just sadness. The feeling of leaving her daughter alone in pain and not knowing when she would be able to come home made Lisa incredibly sad.

Not Wanting To Live Anymore

Mena would express herself and say to her mom, "I'm tired. I just don't want to live anymore. I'm tired of fighting with these doctors and nurses. I'm tired of being in pain. I just feel like I want to die. Nobody understands the pain that I am going through. Nobody understands the way I am feeling. I hate this place. They don't know what they are doing. I'm going to fire my doctor. He doesn't know what he is doing."

Mena recalled hearing someone who was reciting Job with spoken words. Mena felt just like Job 3

It was after this that Job began to speak and to curse the day of his birth. [2] Job said: [3]"Let the day perish on which I was born, also the night when someone said: 'A man has been conceived!' [4] Let that day be darkness. Let God above show no concern for it; Let no light shine upon it. [5] Let the deepest darkness reclaim it. Let a rain cloud settle over it. Let whatever darkens the day terrify it. [6] That night - let the gloom seize it; Let it not rejoice among the days of a year, And let it not enter among the number of the months. [7] Indeed! Let that night become barren; Let no joyful cry be heard in it, [8] Let those who curse the day put a curse on it, Those who are able to awaken Leviathan (crocodile or some other large, powerful aquatic animal) [9] Let the stars of its twilight grow dark; Let it wait in vain for daylight, And let it not see the rays of dawn. [10] For it did not close the doors of my mother's womb; Nor did it hide trouble from my eyes. [11] Why did I not die at birth? Why did I not perish when I came from the womb? [12] Why were there knees to receive me And breasts to nurse me? [13] For now I would be lying down undisturbed; I would be sleeping and at rest ... .[16] Or why was I not like a hidden miscarriage, Like children who have never seen the light? [20] Why does he give light to one who is suffering And life to those in bitter distress? [21] Why do they long for death, but it does not come? They dig for it more than for hidden treasure, [22] Those who are rejoicing greatly, Who are happy when they find the grave. [23] Why does he give light to a man who has lost his way, Whom God has hedged in? [24] For in place of my food comes my sighing, And my groaning pours out like water. [25] For what I have dreaded has come upon me, And what I have feared has befallen me. [26] I have had no peace, no quiet, no rest, But trouble keeps coming." –New World Translation of the Holy Scriptures (Study Edition)

Has this rainy Monday truly gotten Mena down? Mena felt as though she was entering the dark side. She couldn't get out of the water. Rough seas were in sight. She just couldn't catch a break. She wanted to change her name to Mia, which means "My Heart". She needed her heart to be still. She was drowning in the sea of Sickled Cells.

Chapter 19

Everything Coming at Me
From Different Directions
(Snowflakes)

What Are Snowflakes? Each snowflake is made of as many as 200 ice crystals. Some snowflakes are symmetrical, like the type that you cut from paper. They form a hexagonal (six-sided) shape because that is how water molecules organize themselves as they freeze. Some snowflakes become lopsided if they fall sideways to the ground. Snowflakes that spin like tops as they fall to the ground stay symmetrical. https://scied.ucar.edu

Dangerous Falling Snowflakes

Mena felt as if she were in a dream, driving in her car. She could see the snow descending upon her car. She felt as though the car was protecting her from the spears that the snow was shooting at her. It was a beautiful abstract picture that had come to life. The snow was falling from all directions. Vertical, horizontal, diagonal, up and down, all around like a whirlwind. Anxiety began to surge upon her like a roaring lion with no sound. How could she escape this winding road that curved throughout this unwanted journey? The trees bowed downward on both sides of the road, keeping her confined in her car with no way out. She was unable to go left or right on this narrow, winding road. It was cloudy and getting darker and darker. The sun was no longer able to be found. Mena's Sickle Cell had already been interfering with her sight. Most of the time, all she was able to see was blotches of black circles hindering her vision in one eye. Her operation on her eyes was already scheduled, but for now, not even a glimmer of sun rays was shining through to make her pathway straight. No matter how she tried to stop this anxiety, the snow continued to try to break through her windshield. For sure, if the snow penetrated through the windshield, it would cut her like a knife.

The Doctor's Words of Anguish

That's how Mena felt about the doctors' words of anxiety. She could hear the words and voice of the doctor echoing in her ears, stabbing her over and over again from all directions with no help in sight. His words were going against every grain in her body and mind. It was like riding on a winding road, never meeting her designation of releasing her from her pain. He was killing her sharply with his words, trying carefully as a professional not to be sued for what he was saying as a doctor or about what he was planning to do. That was to discharge her with discharged papers.

Hospital Course (Mena's Diagnosis):

The Doctor wrote 44-year-old lady.

Mena's thoughts were in her mind, "Imagine that he sees me as an old lady."

The discharge papers stated with a history of SC(Sickle Cell) disease prior history of AVM and chronic pain who presented with right upper quadrant pain associated with joint pain and right leg pain and was considered to have Sickle Cell crisis treated conservatively with IV fluids and patient HBS 41.3 and reticulocyte count peaked at 2.0, LDL remained within normal parameters and did not require any transfusion and her hemoglobin improved to 10/3/29.3 on day of discharge with improvement in her joint pains and on day of the discharge she reported her pain has improved but still having 5-6/10 in intensity pain but reported that she is feeling better to go home discharge home with recommendations to continue oxycodone 30 mg every 4 hours and for breakthrough pain ordered oxycodone 10 mg every 4 hours 20 tablets and counseled patient to follow-up with PCP and hematologist.

Referrals and Follow-ups to Schedule

AMB REFERRAL TO COMMUNITY HEALTH WORKER

Patient advises that she is having difficulty paying her utility bill and has missed appointments due to a lack of transportation.

"Lies, Lies, Lies," Mena said as she read on, "I have a car of my own, and my family always takes me to the hospital when I need their help. True, I may be behind in my electric bill, but I've got that all handled as well."

Social Determinants Of Health Reasons (PLEASE CHOOSE TOP 3):

Utility Assistance Application

Transportation Application Assistance

Need to know Information: (Covid +, Behavior Issues, Special Needs, etc.): Other Special Needs (Specify in comments) Comment-Sickle Cell

~TODAY YOU WERE REFERRED TO ANOTHER PROVIDER OR FACILITY~

A REFERRAL COORDINATOR WILL CONTACT YOU WITH THE APPOINTMENT DETAILS AND INSTRUCTIONS

On Social Media, Mena expressed how she was feeling after being in the hospital, "Sickle Cell keeps testing me, but I won't let it get the best of me. How do I keep going? Keep fighting this pain that makes me feel insane. My brain stays focused. This too shall pass. My children need me, so I'll fight until I can't anymore. I have so much love to give and so much more in store. The energy from my ancestors and the highest won't let me die. I've got a lot of love left for myself, family, and friends. I'll never give up. I'll never give in. Sickle cell, you lose every time."

Facebook Page Friends

Mena wrote these words on her Facebook page:

"#Sicklecell #fusicklecell #allyouneedislove #sicklecell youlose #warrior #sickecellwarrior"

Mena was not alone in her fight. Her Facebook friends gave her a shout-out!

Facebook Page

{Krystal Njie and 80 others}

Mena had 80 responses on her Facebook social page.

Shonda Robinson, image of a Dove flying with the words Prayers.

Frances Vernique Donaldson-Neal, Be strong, babes!!"

Siobhan Crystal, "Prayers for healing and strength." With three images of purple hearts.

Gwen Morgan, "Prayers for you."

Alicia Shand, "Prayers cuz." Mena responded, "Thank you, beautiful ladies. It won't rain forever."

Missy Smothers, "Get well, sweetheart. You got this." Mena said, "Love you." Missy Smothers, "Love you more."

Krystal Njie, "Sickle Cell can kick rocks! You are so strong! A force unbroken!!!" picture with a fisted arm. Mena answered her, "Thanks, little sis. Love you.

Tara Drayton, "Feel better soon, Warrior," with a heart signal.

Mildred Briscoe, images of praying hands, a heart, praying hands, and a heart. Mena responded to everyone, "Love you guys."

Latisha Nibblett, "Be strong, my beautiful SC disease sister! You are courageous and got this!" images praying hands and a heart. Mena said, "Thanks, beautiful. We all have to link soon."

Anais Jendayi Mennginie, an image of a redheaded girl with her hands in prayer.

Regina Maria Franco Jurado, "Praying for you. And praying they find a cure or at least a treatment that makes living with SC a lot easier." Images of two hearts. Mena gave an answer to that and said, "It should've been done, but you know. At least they're trying to know. Thanks, luv."

Kirston Planter, "Get well soon." With an image of a heart. Mena replied to Kirston, "We got this. I'm glad you're home." Kirston said, "Yes, we do…I'm glad too.

Sabrina Trader, image with a finger rubbing a kitten's chin, saying, "KEEP THAT CHIN UP, FIGHTER!!! YOU GOT THIS!" Mena replied, "always" with a happy emoji.

Amber Mylyfe Mytruth, "Sending you lots of love and prayers." A GIF, with flowers flashing that said, "get well soon."

Shirley Dashiell, "Keep on pushing, Lady! God's got you! Love."

Leslie Parker, "Keep pushing, Mena. I love you."

Annette Christian, "I hope you feel better soon."

Shanda Finney, images of 3 praying hands, two claps, one handmade heart, and an arm fist.

Adedoyin Gloria Ogundehin, "You got this, Sweetheart." Images of a purple heart and praying hands.

Holbrook Rose, an image of "Thinking of you, Sending Love & Hugs FOR BOTH YOU & YOUR MOM." Lisa replied, "Thank You So Much."

Dante Rogers, "Hang in there, cousin."

Eric Briscoe, images of a red heart, two praying hands, and another red heart.

Zyris McCormick, "You got this!!!!" And three arm fists.

Dana McClellan, "Oh no, my beautiful cuzo, I pray you feel better soon. I miss your sweet soul.. sending u lots of prayers n love ur way."

Tiffany Thompson, image of praying hands.

These responses truly lifted Mena's spirit. She was so grateful for her family and friends' comments.

OxyContin out of the question "NOPE"

Mena was going through a rough time with her body. Once again, her body was rejecting everything that entered her stomach. She had been vomiting so much that day that she was getting dehydrated.

Mena picked up the phone and called her mom. Lisa answered, "Hello."

Mena said, "Mom, I have been throwing up all day, and I don't want to go to the hospital."

Lisa said, "It is best that you go just to get some fluids in you. You don't have to stay to get admitted. Just go get some fluids in you."

Mena nauseously said, "I don't want to go right now. There's going to be too many people there, and school has just let out. I will get Mario or Amelia to take me later."

Lisa said, "Okay, but please don't wait too long. If we have to go over the bridge, we need to leave right now, so that we won't be leaving too late."

Lisa was hoping and praying that Mena would be okay because she knew that Mena was going to refuse to be treated at her home hospital. Mena didn't see eye to eye with the doctors and some of the nurses there. Not only does Mena have a distrust for the Hematologist, she would rather die than let him touch her. She felt that he didn't know what he was talking about and that he only cared for the cancer patients. Mena decided to go later that evening, because she wasn't getting any better.

Mena said, "Mom, they have me on fluids but not much for the pain. They tried to put me on OxyContin. Nope, nope, nope. That's the medicine I was on in Fayetteville, and Mrs. Joyce said I looked gray. It's horrible and addictive."

Mrs. Joyce's name means winsomely lovely. She was just that to Mena and her children. Mr. Gregory, which means watchful and Mrs. Joyce, which means whimsomely lovely, friends of Mena's parents, had always been there for Mena and the children. They always looked after them by giving Mena and her children wonderful, cooked meals. Mrs. Joyce would do Mena's girls' hair when Mena was broken down with swollen fingers that she just couldn't do the job.

Mena continued to say, "Also, OxyContin was the medication I took and weaned myself off. It's like glue when it melts. It coats the body inside, which is why it's an extended-release formulation. It's like glue and sticks to your insides. It's funny because I was just talking to the nurse about that."

The doctor entered Mena's room. The doctor said to Mena, "We have ordered OxyContin." Mena said, "The nurse never said that's what you were ordering. She told me something completely different."

Lisa thought about the bad memories of what it used to do to Mena and how she became a different person. It made her strung out. She seemed to be high as a kite, not responding to anything that was going on around her. Lisa had also read about how addictive it can be and how it could affect your organs.

Lisa then asked about the IV fluids, "How is that working for you?"

Mena answered, "It's dripping so slowly. I've had 2 bags so far and I'm starting to feel better."

Lisa was so relieved that Mena was getting out of the woods of sticks and stones of pain. She was also happy to know that she wasn't going to have to take Mena to another hospital that was 2 ½ hours out of town.

Mena Worries About A Way Out

Mena had been so worried about paying her bills. Her rent, electricity, water bill, and phone bill. They were all attacking her at once. She had more money going out than coming in. It was time to make a phone call to her kid's father, Rex. She was determined that she wasn't going to let him get away without helping her with the youngest two kids. He had helped before, and she was determined to get him to help her again. Mena was so stressed out that she paid the same phone bill twice. They wouldn't give it back; they would just credit it to her next bill. That definitely wouldn't help when she needed it back right now for her electricity bill.

Lisa was willing to help, but Mena knew that her mom was retired and was also budgeting their money. Her dad would soon be retiring, and she didn't want to be a burden to them. Mena wasn't thinking about her kids being their grandchildren and that her parents were willing to help out in any way that they could. Lisa knew that Mena was considered disabled and was on a fixed income, so she was motivated to help in any way that she could, especially if it would keep Mena from going into a Sickle Cell Crisis. Mario was on his way to a job interview. Jobs would come and go for him. He had to put college on hold for now to help out his mother. He was like the to-go guy. He would go and take the family, aunts, uncles, and friends anywhere they needed to go. That was his hustle until he could find a decent job. Amelia was in the Army Reserves, working and going to college. She did what she could to help out her mother. It was truly draining on her. However, Amelia often mustered the strength to help take care of her mother and siblings.

This oppressive system was wearing Mena down. She was being hit from all directions, physically, financially, and socially. Lack of money, bills, dealing with the hospital, ex-husband, and lies. Like the falling icy snow, which takes no mercy, hitting you with its sharpness and stinging feeling. Mena thought to herself, would she fall on her face with the feeling of falling on hard, impacted snow on a cold surface? The snow was getting deeper, and so were her bills. The bill collectors would show no mercy. It would be as if Mena was in a ground blizzard, being hit smack in the face, giving her no visibility in sight. Where would she go, and whom should she turn to, not knowing where to turn?

Chapter 20

People Are Staying Here Too Long (Animal Control)

Animal control—An animal control service or animal control agency is an entity charged with responding to requests for help with animals, including wild animals, dangerous animals, and animals in distress. Wikipedia. What is the meaning of animal control? An office or department responsible for enforcing ordinances relating to the control, impoundment, and disposition of animals.

https://www.merriam-webster.com Is animal control state or local? Is animal control state or local? Animal control and animal sheltering are government responsibilities, so local officials decide if these services will be provided by a government agency or contractor unless law or charter provisions determine the decision. https://www.alleycat.org

Mena was in the kitchen, enjoying the moment of playing with her cats. Her cell phone rang. It was Precious, Mena's friend. She needed someone to talk to, and she knew that Mena had been an advocate for her so many times when she was in the hospital. Precious was so distraught after having a conversation with the Hematologist and a nurse who treated her as if she had no value at all. Precious name means "of great worth" or "highly esteemed." It also meant a reminder of love and adoration. The Hematologist and Nurse truly knocked Precious' name out of the window. The conversation in the room between Mena's friend, the Hematologist, and the nurse was daunting.

We're Not Doing That Anymore

The doctor came in already with a chip on his shoulder and said, "Ahhhhhh, for those people who feel that they have to have Dilaudid, ahh then maybe some other hospital will give it, but we're, we're not giving it. Okay, just so you know that."

Precious responded, "Oh."

In the middle of the Hematologist's persistent talk. The Hematologist went on in his speech, "Just so you know that, cause you've been admitted before. When we were giving morphine and you were fine, you know. When we didn't have Dilaudid."

Precious answered him by saying, "Yeah, but I feel it took longer to get over the hard part with just the morphine."

The hematologist talks over her and says, "Yeah, but this is what we are going to stick with. You know we have people staying toooo long. You know when they are getting Dilaudid. We're not going to do that anymore."

Well, Mena was listening to Precious' side of the story, she interrupted her and said to Precious, "They aren't treating us like patients. They are treating us like problems to be managed. Like animals staying in a shelter."

Precious nodded her head and agreed. Precious went on with her story.

The hematologist said, "Alright! So, we are only giving it under special circumstances. If you hear that somebody else is getting it, that's their business. I don't know what they're doing. We're not, we're not doing this, on this, on this floor anymore. Okay,"

Precious replied, "Oh, yeah."

The doctor said, "Alright, alright."

The nurse entered the floor and said, "Hello, Hi."

Precious says, "Hi."

The nurse said to the Hematologist, "Precious had called Condition H earlier when I was here."

As the nurse entered, it was as if she was responsible for enforcing ordinances relating to the control of the disposition of Precious.

The hematologist said, "Right, I'm talking to her about the Dilaudid. We're not giving her Dilaudid as we used to. That's our new rule, okay, especially for the Sicklers."

Sicklers

Precious mind was wandering off, thinking to herself, "Whose rule is this anyway, the State or Federal, they are treating me like I'm under animal control?"

The doctor went on to say, "In the old days, we would have Sicklers stay in for two weeks and get their Dilaudid. I remember when you were here. When we stopped having it, we suddenly didn't see people here. Okay, we're giving morphine. They'd come in, they wouldn't stay as long as they used to."

Racing in Precious' mind was the thought that the hematologist acted as if he were part of a control agency to stop the overstay of Sickle Cell Patients like animals in distress.

The hematologist slowly said, "We're not going to give Dilaudid again unless it's a very special circumstance."

Precious responded, "I know what you're saying, but I'm not just, you can't put me in the same category with everybody."

Precious started speaking to herself, "Who decides if these services would be provided by the hospital or a governmental agency? Who makes these decisions?"

The Hematologist answered her category question, "Well, I've watched you since you came to this admission, so I know how you are now compared to the way you were when you first came. You're not in as much pain as when you first came."

Precious said, in a nervous state barely able to get her correct wording out, "But okay, I mean okay, well it's really no need to talk about it, if okay you're saying, if you're not giving it, okay we can just leave it. I mean."

The Hematologist interrupted once again, "Well, that's, that's, yeah, that's basically it. I just wanted to come here myself to let you know, okay."

Precious said in defeat, "Yeah."

The hematologist said, "Yeah."

The nurse said, "Yeah, because we had, we had talked about it. I know she had said she was on her pain medicine, her POP medicine at home. We had even talked about possibly trying to see if she could start switching to that to see how she'll do at home."

While the nurse was talking, the hematologist interrupted her before she could finish what she was saying.

The Hematologist said, "Yeah, we could switch to that, the POP medicine."

The nurse proceeded to say more, talking to Precious and the hematologist, "Because we had even talked about it, she does get POP Dilaudid at home, right, Precious? Isn't that what you get at home? But I don't know if she is receptive to that or not."

The Hematologist was still talking over the nurse, stating, "We could switch it to PO Dilaudid, but no IV Dilaudid. Not Going to Happen, Yeah."

The nurse continued, "I also tried to explain that 6 mgs of morphine is a higher dose. I understand that Sicklers are in or have pain. These are all the interesting things we talk about."

As the nurse spoke, she gestured, moving her arm in a circular motion. Then she folded her hands back, one over the other, in front of her white-coated body, standing straight and tall, staring and talking as Precious lay nervously in the bed. "Um, I tried to help her understand all that."

Conversation We Are Having Now

Precious finally spoke up, stumbling in her words and said, "I mean, I was just; I mean, I feel like, it just was you know, I used to have it and then it would just stop all of a sudden. I feel like this conversation should have been had when it first happened anyway."

In such a smart way, the Hematologist replied, "Well, we're having it now."

Precious attacked back nervously, "Well, we could have prevented all this."

The Hematologist once again said, "We're having it now. This conversation…"

Precious then said, "It wouldn't even be, it wouldn't even be a subject right now. I mean, I feel like if something helps, that, that's what I would want to stick with, but I mean I can't control what kind of rules, yeah, have right now."

Precious proceeded to roll her feet and move them side to side in an upset, nervous way, in and out of the covers.

The hematologist replied, "All right, okay, so I've let you know. All right. Hopefully, you'll be better soon to go home, because you are much, much better than when you first came in. Okay, we need to start the ball rolling for going home."

"Thanks," the nurse says, "Okay, all right."

The monitor suddenly started beeping loudly as if to say this conversation was over. The conversation took four minutes and fifteen seconds. The Hematologist had his way.

Precious said to Mena, "I had no one to eradicate for me."

Precious thought once again to herself, "What is a Sickler? Did the Hematologist and the nurse respond to her request for help?" Throughout this whole conversation, who in the hell was We? Who was making up the rules?"

Not Happening

Two weeks later, Mena found herself in the same position. Same floor. Same feeling: "nobody's listening." The same hematologist argued about giving her Dilaudid when she needed it. When the hematologist finally decided to give her the Dilaudid, it would only be in a pill form. Mena argued against this because she had never been given Dilaudid in this form. She had refused to take it. She argued with the doctor, stating what they were trying to do to her. Why make a change in a pill form? They had always given her Dilaudid through an IV? If it ain't broke, don't try to fix it.

Mena was feeling the same way Precious was feeling. She felt like if something helped, she would like to stick to it. Mena stood her ground and refused to take it in pill form. No matter how bad the pain was.

Mena called her mother, Lisa, about the situation. Lisa had gotten nowhere speaking to the Supervisor Nurse. She said, "Nothing is going to change about the decision the doctor had made in the hospital. The Dilaudid was still going to be given in pill form. So, Lisa decided to contact the NAACP about what was happening with her daughter and other Sickle Cell patients in the hospital. This was something new and mind-boggling to Mena and Lisa. They would just wait to hear from the NAACP and Wanda, who was in charge of organizing community walks for the town where they lived, for those affected by Sickle Cell disease and their families. Wanda's mother named her that because she felt that one day Wanda would be a shepherdess. She would defend the community in some way. She would be a symbol of courage. Mena and Lisa needed help. They were just getting nowhere on their own.

Mena had received an exchange of blood. Mena knew that Lisa would talk to her later, because she knew her mother would never agree to that procedure. Lisa had read that having too many blood exchanges can lead to significant health problems. Damage to the organs, immune reaction, allergic reactions and the transfused white blood cell could attack Mena. Mena's hemoglobin had been at an 8, and finally, it climbed to a 10. There seemed to be a string of hope coming that Mena would be coming back home soon to her family.

Overstayed Welcome

I'm sure the doctors and nurses felt as though Mena had overstayed her welcome in the hospital. When that happens with animals in a shelter, sometimes they have to be put to sleep, but fortunately for Mena's sake, that was not the case. It was illegal to put a patient to sleep. Usually, the patients will decide for themselves to leave or they will call the security guard to escort them out. It's like being put back out on the street with no shelter to ease their pain. Mena was a fighter not just for herself but for the other Sickle Cell patients. She would be strong and not let them cause her to go astray, but hang right in there until she knew she could tolerate her pain level and that her hemoglobin levels were where they needed to be. Mena would need a tub soaking and a massage. Well, that's what Lisa would want anyway.

Once again, Mena felt as if "Nobody's listening to Me." The day was winding down, and Mena would rest up. That's if it were possible between the pain and lack of sleep. Preparing for another day to fight and to express herself, she thought once again, "If Only They Could See Me."

Mena had a fairly good memory for reading topics about Sickle Cell. There was an article on the Johns Hopkins page, "The Thorny History of Sickle Cell." The Quote was:

"ONE THING WE'RE SEEING IS THAT A LOT OF THINGS ABOUT SICKLE CELL DISEASE HAVE NOT CHANGED. IT'S STILL A RACIALIZED DISEASE. IT'S STILL A DISEASE WITH TREMENDOUS HEALTH CARE DISPARITIES." -Lydia Pecker. Mena also remembered her being the Director of the Young Adult Clinic in the Johns Hopkins Sickle Cell Center for Adults. Mena thought about the definition of disparities.

Disparities: a difference in level or treatment, especially one that is seen as unfair.

This chapter is in memory of Precious. Precious died at her home. She succumbed to this deadly disease at the age of 46. Precious didn't look her age. She still looked like a teenager whose age hadn't caught up with her. Mena had discovered, in the darkness of Social Media, which had now surfaced into the light. Mena cried profusely upon hearing this news about her dear friend, who had struggled to advocate for herself at times. Mena's memory of Precious was of her beautiful brown eyes, her long braided hair, and her pink, rosy lips. Precious fought for her life, her voice, and her dignity. But the system didn't listen. Now it was up to Mena and all those who loved her to ensure that all Precious's hopes and dreams were not in vain. Mena wanted to make sure that Precious' voice echoed long after she was gone, and others who had fought the fine fight.

Chapter 21

Misfit (Shrub Rose)

Shrub Roses have characteristics that others do not, and yet they are beautiful. A shrub is any plant that is woody and has multiple stems. Classification means it does not fit within all the categories. Saying it is defined by what it's not. They're not right for the other categories. These are not climbers. There is not a single rule. Shrubs are not in a certain class. Hybrid Musk is large and loose. The David Alton Rose should not be dumped ceremoniously into shrubs. The David Alston Rose is one of the most successful breeding program roses in human history, and everything that is distinct about these roses. They should be revisited. Politics situation. Some roses have the same shape, size, and look. http://www.fraservalleyrosefarm.com

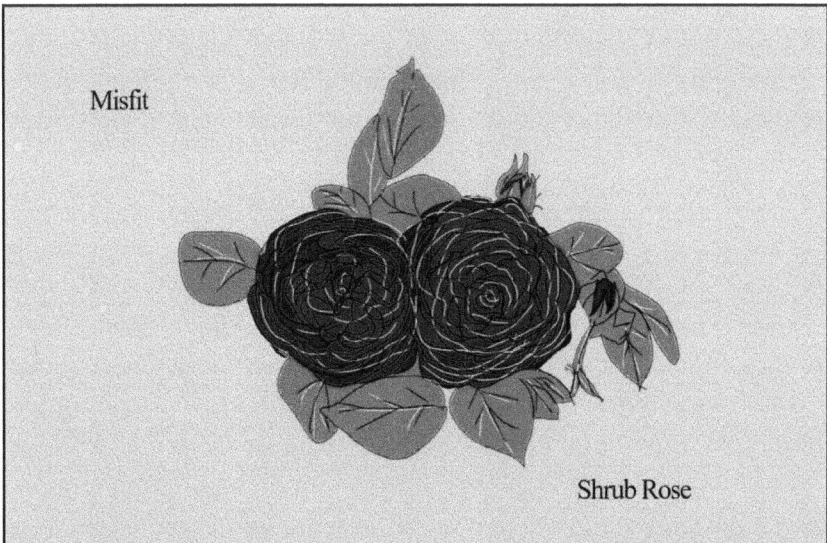

Misfit

Shrub Rose

Don't Care To Fit In

Mena thought to herself, *"Oh, you Sickled Cells. My body is not like a keyhole where you can unlock it and just come in. I did not leave a light on for you to enter my body to cause mass destruction."*

Mena's heart was racing fast, and her liver and spleen were enlarged as well. Just to mention, Mena's hemoglobin was 11-12 when she came into the hospital. Now it's 7-8.

Her attitude and behavior set her apart from others, and that is why Mena started talking to herself, saying, "The doctors don't see me for who I am. They see me as an outcast. Someone who is seeking drugs."

Mena saw herself as being brilliant, knowledgeable, assertive, and persistent. She felt as though she could be like an owl going in both directions. Being positive about self-enhancement, she could also be self-effacing, demanding, arrogant, and extremely outspoken. She wanted to stay out of the spotlight and not even be noticed. She could be like a light bulb turning on and off.

Mena went on talking to herself, "To be honest, I don't care if I fit in or not."

She was always trying to remove herself from various situations, like arguing with the doctors and nurses.

Mena carried on with the conversation to herself. "It doesn't make me an unhappy person because I believe in myself, and I am greatly confident I am a strong woman."

The suffering Mena was feeling was that this disease was causing her to be nauseated. Her arms, legs, and hips hurt, and her hands and ankles were swollen. She had done her research about this awful disease. She knew that she could tell the doctors what her body needed. She could tell them the several types of Sickle Cell. She had caused them to feel embarrassed because of their lack of knowledge. The doctors and nurses had come to feel ashamed. Mena knew that they didn't like her because they didn't smile at her, and they avoided eye contact.

Mena said to herself, "They gossip about me, they talk about me, and most of all, they don't C me, they try to ignore me. Nobody's listening. It's as if they are defining me as something that I am not."

A song entered Mena's mind about the doctors and nurses, "Oh, here she comes, she's a man-eater…" by Daryl Hall & John Oates. Mena sang "Oh, here they come, they are mind eaters, watch out!"

The Discharged Papers From The Emergency Room

Mike, the hospital administrator, stepped into the room with a stack of discharge papers. His face said it all–he wasn't here to help.

Mena's fist clenched under the blanket. Her voice cracked as she said, "I'm not a drug seeker. I just want to live."

Mena spoke aloud, "You think I'm a drug seeker. I can do that at home. I don't have anything in my system right now. Now I have to start all over again with my meds." She went on to address Mike, the hospital administrator, "My Hemoglobin is seven. What are you comparing a nine to? My levels are normally eleven to twelve. I was in pain when my hemoglobin level was at ten. I am not a drug seeker. I don't like the way any drugs make me feel. I have kids at home. Pain for me may not be pain for you. Yes, I fell asleep on the bathroom toilet. My body is exhausted. The Phenergan you gave me makes me sleepy. I haven't slept in two days because of the pain. My breathing is low, and my heart rate is low."

Mike replied, "They are scientists. We have compared your numbers with those from your previous doctor's lab work, and your numbers appear to be fine. There is no point in admitting you to the hospital. Doctor Mills says that he isn't giving you anymore."

Mena asked, "What about the doctors in the emergency room notes?"

Mike, the administrator, answered her by saying, "The Emergency Room doctors are not going to get involved in your case. There is really very little we can do. You have seen two providers. We are running out of options. Both doctors concur."

Mike went on to say, "I understand where you're coming from. At this point and time, you need to seek another institution; VCU has grants."

Mena answered them by saying in a frustrated voice, "What's the purpose?"

Mike said, "I have little to offer at this point. Here are your discharge instructions on what to do at home. I'm sorry."

Mena felt as though her demeanor and the way she was feeling had reached a point of no return. She said, "I am trying to live a healthy life. Sorry, it doesn't help anything. No one has bothered to call VCU. It's okay. I know the doctors are lying because I called VCU, where my doctor is located. Their office said that no one from here has spoken to my doctor there. You all lied to me. Every single time I come here, I am treated like crap, as if I were a misfit, as if I don't belong here. You shouldn't be labeling anyone like that. My charge nurse, Tammy, who looked like a palm tree, because of her hair, wouldn't even tell me her last name."

Mena begins to cry profusely. "I wish you could feel a glimpse of how I am feeling."

Mike said, "They said it was 5 hours ago that they took your blood. Just repeat Benadryl and Toradol, which is a little stronger than Motrin. I am 100% sure they won't run any more blood work. It's not changing just that fast."

Fighting For Medical Care

Mena gave her attention back to her mother after Mike left. "Mommy, I tried to come to this hospital to get help. They just don't get it. I wish they could feel what I feel right now. They talked amongst each other, deciphering what to do with me. Do you think they care? No, they don't care. Nobody's listening to me. If only they could C me. They gave me medication that made me sleepy. I fell asleep on the toilet. I was drained from lack of sleep and the meds. They didn't even tell me they took the monitor off. Let someone come in with a migraine, and see if they wouldn't help them. They keep giving me mixed signals. They kept acting like I was displeasing them. They kept coming like they were displeased, huffing and puffing. My arms, legs, and hips are paining me. I've been in pain all day. I feel nauseous. All the doctors did was shake their heads. Ma Mi I am so tired of having Sickle Cell. Mommy, I must repeat how I am feeling. Nobody's listening to me. If only they could C me."

Lisa heard her repeating the same phrases over and over again. This was truly how Mena was feeling. Lisa said, "Why don't we try another hospital?"

Mena replied with extreme sadness, "Virginia is four hours away. No one cares."

You could hear the defeat of agony in her voice. Mena just bowed her head down, for she had lost the battle for now, but not the war. All the knowledge she had displayed and talked about that day hadn't paid off. She was still a misfit to them. Just like the shrub rose she just didn't fit in. They couldn't place her in any category. Those were Mena's feelings. She was in a moment of shedding tears. Her tears were about to come out at any moment once again; she was defined by what she was not.

Lisa was listening to the whole conversation on the phone and taking notes. She was very distraught by every word that she had heard. It was a shame that her daughter was fighting for a cause, fighting for her life. The doctors and the Patient Advocacy for Mena were definitely not comforters for Mena. Lisa read the Bible often, and it reminded her of a situation that Job was in. He stood up for himself against the three comforters who were supposed to be his friends, but instead, they were no comforters at all. Job had said:

Job: 7:9-11

Like a cloud that fades and vanishes,

The one who goes down to the

Grave does not come back up,

He will not return again to his house,

And his place will acknowledge him no more.

Therefore, I will not restrain my mouth.

I will speak in the anguish of my spirit:

I will complain in my bitter distress!

Mena thought about shrub roses. No matter how beautiful shrub roses are, some feel that they are not right for certain categories. I know that's how some doctors feel about those who have Sickle Cell. Some doctors can not see the beauty that lies within them. They feel as if Sickle Cell Patients are not in the right category like cancer patients, even though there are some connections and similarities between the two conditions. Sickle Cell can be defined by what it's not. That's why some doctors say some types of Sickle Cell are milder than others. That's not the case for all. Both, however, do involve the blood cells. For example, Leukemia involves uncontrolled cell division, and Sickle Cell is an abnormality in the red blood cells. Why should cancer patients be given more attention in cures and funding? Is this a political situation? Maybe so.

Mena voiced herself, "There are unprofessional doctors everywhere, but don't let them shut you up. Your voice matters. Mine does too. Even if nobody's listening–I'll keep speaking. Please, don't let them silence you."

Chapter 22

Mommy and Daughter Talk (Sulcata African Spurred Tortoise)

Tortoises love 70 degrees or over during the day and can stay outside if the temperature stays above 50 at night. They will get enough natural sunlight, which is important for Vitamin D, and they can eat grass and other plants. They can barge through anything in their way, so heavy reinforcement is necessary. They are very sociable with people, gentle, and intelligent. They have a long lifespan of 100 years. They will seek out their owners for positive interaction. They have to be willed to family members. https://www.denherdervet.com They walk at a speed of 0.13 to 0.30 mph. Tortoises are notoriously slow. The shell is the tortoise's main protection. The most widely accepted hypotheses regarding the longevity of turtles relate to their slow metabolism. https://naturemuseum.org

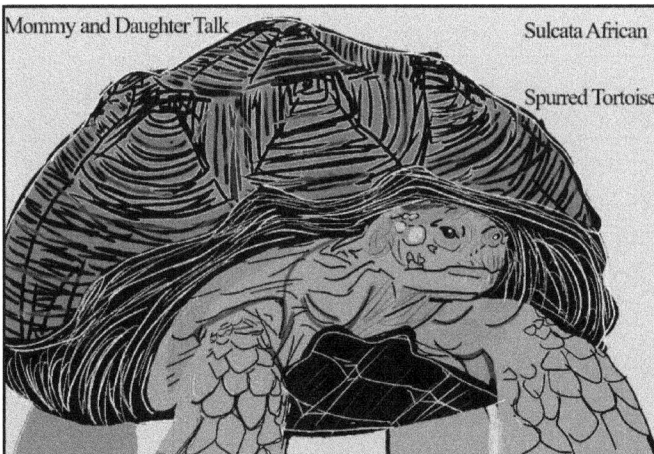

Mommy and Daughter Talk — Sulcata African Spurred Tortoise

Lisa's Bonding Visit

Lisa was on pins and needles going for a visit to see her daughter. She didn't know if her daughter would be in a good mood or a bad mood. Lisa just knew that she wanted her and her daughter to talk to each other in a civilized manner. This time, she wasn't going to make this a rushed visit with other things to do. The Sulcata African Spurred Tortoise is known for its slowness. Mena was slow in everything that she did. She hated people who rushed her. Lisa could see the slowness in Mena. It was as if she was watching her move in slow motion.

Mena was never on time for anything. On Lisa's last visit, Mena said, "If you're going to be in a hurry or you have things to do, then just don't come at all."

Lisa wondered if Mena's slowness brought her longevity. Would Mena's youthful years beat the odds of Mena's life being cut short? The Tortoise is known for wanting positive interaction. That is just what Mena and Lisa wanted. Lisa was sociable with others, but she needed to work on that with her daughter. Mena, on the other hand, when she wasn't well, she didn't display a sociable quality. When she was in pain, she would rather be left alone. Lisa was gentle and kind in trying to phrase her words with Mena, but somehow, Mena's intelligent quality, which allowed her to know so much about things, would always get in the way. Mena was like the tortoise; she would barge through anything that was getting in her way.

She would say, "This is how I am, and I'm not changing for anyone. You either like me or you don't, and if you don't, then get out of my way."

In Lisa's mind, sometimes she wanted to do just that, not get in Mena's way! Today was not the day for getting in Mena's way. This was going to be a bonding visit. Lisa had neglected to hear Mena's side of the story about her condition for years. Lisa had read about Sickle Cell disease from time to time; however, it was never serious reading, just the fundamental information about it.

Mena's words had slapped her in the face when Mena had said to her, "You don't have to come and visit me, I am used to being alone."

Lisa never wanted to ever hear her daughter say those words again. Lisa felt ashamed of herself for not really being there for Mena. Lisa always felt that Mena's husband and friends would come and visit Mena a lot, so Lisa thought that Mena was never lonely. In Lisa's defense, Mena hadn't been home in the past 6 years anyway. Lisa felt that now she had no excuse for not being there for Mena, considering she lives in the same town. Mena had been home for three years now, and Lisa was very seldom there for Mena while she was in the hospital. She was busy working, being a housewife, and managing her ministry, as well as watching Mena's kids in her absence. This visit was going to be special. She didn't want to hear Mena say those words, "Nobody's Listening to Me" or "Mom just listen." Lisa decided that she would truly be patient this time. Lisa thought the hard stubbornness in Mena was a protection like the hard shell that protected the tortoise. Mena had built a hard shell around her. Lisa sat back and thought about why Mena was the way she was. Mena could be gentle and sociable when surrounded by her friends or when she felt like herself. She was even kind to the staff if they followed her needs and wants in every way.

Understanding The Different Types of Terminology of Sickle Cell

Lisa entered the room smiling. "Here I go! Hi, Mena, how are you feeling today?"

Mena seemed to be in a great mood. "Feeling better."

That's good to hear. Lisa knew that if she started her conversation off about Sickle Cell, Mena would perk right up. Lisa said to Mena, "I have lots of time to spend with you, let's just have a mommy-daughter talk. I have a few questions about your Sickle Cell. I want to know the difference between Sickle Cell Anemia, which is SS, and HbSC, which is sometimes called Sickle Cell Hemoglobin C disease.Can you help me understand it?"

Mena replied, "Okay, so what I'm going to do is, I'm gonna read it to you to explain it, so that you can understand it better."

Lisa interrupted, "No, I like how you say it."

Mena interrupted, "No, I'm going to explain it like that, just give me a second. I'm going to read to you what they say Sickle Cell Hemoglobin C disease is."

Lisa quickly said, "Okay." She remembered that she was going to be patient and listen. She wasn't going to let this visit turn into a fight. She was going to leave happy and satisfied, and also leave her daughter happy.

Mena read on: "It says people who have Sickle Cell Hemoglobin C disease have red blood cells that contain mostly hemoglobin C. Too much hemoglobin C can reduce the number and size of red blood cells in your body, causing mild anemia."

Lisa said, "I got that." Lisa wanted Mena to know that she was truly listening.

"Okay, so the way I explain it is that when you have Sickle Cell Hemoglobin C disease, a person inherits one sickle Cell gene, and one hemoglobin C gene. Combined, you have S blood cells which would be your Sickle C shape cells or crescent moons as I call it, and you have your Hemoglobin C cells which as I read before has more hemoglobin C that causes you to be anemic, but they are smaller in size. So, you have two types of red blood cells that are working against you. So, when my Hemoglobin drops, it makes me become more anemic. When someone has Sickle Cell, which is SS, they inherit a sickle cell gene (hemoglobin S) from both parents. Their Hemoglobin is already low, which is why they develop anemia behind it. They say Sickle Cell Anemia because they are always anemic. Mine usually sits at 12 and 13, which is very good for someone with Sickle Cell hemoglobin C disease. Often, doctors get it wrong, stating that Sickle Cell is a milder form. I mean, Sickle Cell Hemoglobin C disease is a milder form of Sickle Cell, but I am living proof that's not always true." Mena began to laugh a little, "That, that is not the case. Um, it seems as if my cousin and I have switched rows. Autumn was in the hospital all the time when she was a child, and I wasn't in the hospital all the time when I was a child, so I was able to go swimming and do sports. I ran track, and I did cheerleading. Anything that pushes you to the limit. I like to play football, baseball, and everything. Whereas in Autumn she couldn't do those things, that's because she was anemic. Which you always know, when you're anemic, you're colder a lot of the time. So, when you get into a cold swimming pool, your body is already anemic, which causes it to become even more anemic, leading to a Sickle Cell Crisis, when you have SS. Whereas with Hemoglobin C, we aren't that anemic because our Hemoglobin is better. So, we tend to be able to go swimming and do things like that. Now, as I've gotten older, my Sickle Crisis has gotten worse, whereas Autumn's has kind of, you know, slacked off. She's not in the hospital as frequently as I am. Um, I did have a partial Hysterectomy, which helped with me going to the hospital once a month because of my menstrual cycle. Now, I don't have to go to the hospital once a month. I went to the hospital when I was only bleeding."

Lisa said, "Why is that?" Mena replied, "When you lose blood, you become anemic, losing blood."

Mena took the time to laugh again. Lisa was feeling good to see her daughter laugh. Mena's mood swings can sometimes drive her crazy, but this right here was okay. Her daughter was in a good mood and happy. That meant that Mena was getting better.

Mena continued, "So that is why my crisis has gone down. Thus, when my Hemoglobin drops to eleven, ten, I'm in a crisis, even though it may not look like it to the doctors, as I'm having a crisis, just because my Hemoglobin is good, they're not looking at the fact that I have Sickle Cell hemoglobin C disease. Which is why my Hemoglobin is higher than someone who would have SS."

Sickle Cell Development In Babies

Lisa replied, "Right. So, I also read that when babies are born, they have this protection with their cells."

Mena said, "Fetal Hemoglobin." It's the oxygen carrying protein that is found in the developing fetus. It's there for a few months after birth. Gradually, it takes 6 months to a year for the baby's hemoglobin to turn into adult hemoglobin.

Lisa said, "Yeah, It protects the red blood cells from sickling. So, as the person grows their levels decrease, then symptoms of sickle cell diesease begins to emerge." Lisa then said, "Autumn told me about that."

Mena jumped right in, Fetal Hemoglobin is found in the blood of the umbilical cord."

"What is Fetal Hemoglobin again?"

Nurse Jennifer said, "Cord Blood." Her name means fairness and gentleness. Mena loved her nurse. She was always ensuring that Mena was treated fairly when the others were trying to speak against her. She always made sure that things were going right for Mena. Her words were always gentle and kind, like the sounds of a white surging wave. Mena loved the sound of her voice.

Mena went on with the conversation, "Because you have your fetal Hemoglobin(HbF) in it, and that also helps with stem cells. It's the main protein that carries oxygen in a fetus's red blood cells. It's essential for the fetus to receive enough oxygen from the mother. If you want to get a stem cell transplant, you have to save your cord, your blood cord, I mean your cord blood."

Mena started laughing again because of getting mixed up with Cord Blood. She finished up the Cord Blood information. "Um, you can use that for Stem Cell Transplant, which has helped people get rid of Sickle Cell."

Nurse Jennifer interrupted again and said, "So, why don't everybody do it then?"

The Boy Who Had A Bone Marrow Transplant

Mena said, "I don't know, there was one boy who used to come here who got that procedure done, and he's in remission now from Sickle Cell. I forgot what his name was. He spoke at a college." She sounded as if she was singing the words 'College.' "He was like a trial person. It's so hard, like you're going to die (she sang the words "die out"), like you can die from having a stem cell transplant. It can be complex and a high risk procedure. The donor's immune cells can attack your body."

Lisa remembered reading somewhere that the cost of a bone marrow transplant for Sickle Cell disease was about $200,000 to $400,000. That was stated in statnews.com. That's definitely one of the reasons Sickle Cell patients don't undergo this procedure. Lisa didn't say that reason out loud, because she didn't want to discourage Mena.

Then Jennifer said, "That's what I thought. It's very risky because they arbitrate your immune system pretty much so that your body doesn't reject any of the new cells."

More Meds

Just like that, the conversation changed. Jennifer said, "I gave you some more of your meds, Mena. I don't have anything else. What else do you want?"

Mena answered her by saying, "My stomach is hurting badly."

Jennifer said, "Well, like what else do you want?"

Mena replied, "I don't know, you got something like, I don't know, it just feels like I'm going to throw up (in a low voice) one way or the other."

Jennifer said, "You want like Compazine or something?"

Mena asked, "What's Compazine?" Jennifer replied, "Compazine is like Zofran; it just works in a different way."

Mena said, "Okay."

Jennifer recanted, "But that's not going to make you poop. I would go for the Zofran first and see if you can poop. I would walk around some too that will help you poop."

Mena replied, "I was doing like this in the bathroom if you rock back and forth."

Jennifer asked, "Well, did you stop rocking?"

Mena said, "I didn't stop it."

Lisa was intrigued by the past topic they were talking about. She'd rather not hear about pooping or not pooping. That was a stinky conversation and personal.

Jennifer asked, "So, in a nutshell, if you have SS, what is the percentage of Sickled Cells when you have Sickle Cell Anemia?"

Mena had to think about the answer, so she paused and said, "That one I want to say is 100%, but I know it's not. Hold on…" Mena looked at her cell phone, asking Google out loud, "What percent of Sickle Cell is in a person with Sickle Cell Anemia? It just says a high percentage. The exact percentage can vary."

Blood Exchange

Lisa was changing the conversation they were having all together. I wanted you to also explain to me when you said, um on the phone, the 50, 40."

Mena said, "Oh, with my body? Okay, I'm going to bring that up, so that I can give you the exact numbers."

Lisa said, "Yes, because I remembered you said that your Sickled Cells were like 50% and the Hemoglobin was like 40% that's why you had to get a Blood Transfusion."

Mena interrupted, "I didn't really have any normal Blood Cells. My Sickle Cell, my S's was 50-something percent, and my C's were 40-something percent. So, it was a very small margin of regular Red Blood Cells. That's why I had to have the blood exchange, not a blood transfusion. A Blood Exchange, that's where they take your blood out and then they put some new blood in to try to raise it, to get you some normal, um, Hemoglobin in there."

Lisa asked again to make sure, "So, the C is considered what?"

Mena answered, "A genetic defect." It alters the way the hemoglobin molecule is supposed to be structured.

Then Lisa asked, " So, what is Hemoglobin C disease?"

Mena answered, "Hemoglobin C disease. It's an inherited blood disorder. It affects your hemoglobin protein in the red blood cells. They don't live as long, they are smaller um, and they cause anemia."

Lisa said, "And the S was sickled."

Mena agreed, "Yes, they're sickled, they're sticky, they're hard."

Lisa then said, "So you had Sickle going on."

Mena interrupted, "Disease."

Lisa continued, "And you had tiny little cells like whole cells, little, tiny ones, so you didn't really have any whole blood cells as far as the normal size."

Mena agreed, "Right, I didn't have any normal size uh, Hemoglobin. I just had messed up Hemoglobin."

Delivery of Oxygen

Lisa asked another question. "And the definition of Hemoglobin?"

Mena answered willingly, "The definition of Hemoglobin is the protein contained in red blood cells of vertebrates that is responsible for the delivery of oxygen to the tissues, and that's why a lot of times when your Hemoglobin drops, they are supposed to put you on oxygen."

Lisa replied, "Then if you don't have any oxygen going to the brain, it can cause strokes, heart attacks, and even death."

Mena wholeheartedly agreed and said, "Yes, all of that. You can even have Sickle Cell Crises anywhere that has blood. So, you can have a crisis in your eye, you can have a crisis in your brain. Like you said, a stroke. You can have a crisis in your heart, which causes you to go into cardiac arrest, and the more crisis you have in that same area, the more destruction it does, and that is why I have (AVN) in my shoulder, which is a vascular necrosis, which is bone death. Once your bone starts dying, there is nothing you can do about it, but get a replacement."

Measuring The Volume of The Blood Cells is So Confusing

There was another thing that Lisa was very much concerned about, so she asked this question. "So, being that you keep having a lot of pain in your side...."

Mena just remembered something, so she said, "Oh, one second."

"You asked about the hematocrits. The hematocrits measure the volume of red blood cells compared to "excuse me."

Mena burped.

"Compared to the total blood volume, red blood cells, and plasma.

That's what that is. The normal hematocrit range for men is 40% to 54%, and for women, it is 36% to 48%. This volume can be determined directly by microhematocrit configurations or calculated indirectly. Automated cells counter calculate the hematocrit by multiplying the red cell number in millions by MM3."

Even though Mena was knowledgeable about her Sickle Cell, she admitted and said, "I don't know what that is. By means of cell volume MCV and ventilators. Cheez, that's really, that's crazy. Subject to the vicariates inherent to obtaining an accurate measurement of the MCV."

Lisa was so confused and started to get bored with all the calculation stuff. It meant nothing to her. So, finally, she interrupted and said, "What is MCV?"

Mena signed. "MCV." Lisa was observing that two papers were lying on the table, and she said, "That stayed the same on both papers the MCV."

Mena said, "Yeah, I mean that it's just all the total for like, what you get out of your hematocrit, that's how you get your levels for your hematocrit."

Lisa said, "What's the definition of Hematocrit?" As if she wasn't listening the first time.

Mena replied in frustration, "I just said it." Lisa laughed, "All that long stuff you just said, they need to break that stuff down."

Lisa continued to laugh.

Mena said, "All it is, all it is, is measuring the volume of red blood cells compared to the total blood volume. That's basically what it is."

Lisa said, "Oh, okay."

On to another subject, Mena went. "The blood cells and plasma."

White Blood Cells Gushing Out Of A Boy's Head

Lisa began to think about how late it was getting, now that it was daylight saving time, and she wanted to get home before it was dark. She decided to let Mena go on with all the information she had stored up in her brain. "'Cause you know you have plasma."

Lisa interrupted without thinking, "A type of blood."

Lisa had forgotten how Mena hated it when someone interrupted her before she could get out all she wanted to say. Mena would always say, "Let me finish."

Mena continued, "It's, it's everything that is in your blood. You know that's what's in your blood. As a matter of fact, I saw some plasma come out of this boy's head when I was in elementary school. It looked like white blood cells. I don't know, but he busted his head open and pretty badly; he was just leaking, and all you saw was all this stuff inside of his blood. Y'all."

Lisa cringed at the sight of it in her mind and said, "Ell."

Mena said, "I didn't tell you about that?"

Lisa said, "No. How in the world did he hit his head?"

Mena said, "They were racing and the bars were uneven bars, but you know how the bars go down and go down."

Lisa said, "The single bars?"

Mena, "Yes, the single bars, and then they have the lower single bars. They were racing, and the one boy went like that, but he didn't bend over to go underneath the bar, and he was running extremely fast. He was so fast that when he hit the bar, he busted his head open, and all of a sudden, the teachers were screaming, and you look, and it was just leaking. It's just pouring out like somebody's pouring a glass of water. It was just leaking out."

Lisa asked, "Oh my goodness, did he survive?"

Mena said, "Y'all, he lived, but it was something I will never forget. Then, he came back with a T on his head, where they had to suture his head back up. He went to the hospital, I guess, where it was a good facility. This hospital was never good because when I came to this hospital, they didn't know what was wrong with me. And the hospital that I am talking about is _____."

Lisa quickly interrupted the bad language Mena was about to use. Then Mena proceeded to name the city and zip code. "Just in case anyone wants to know."

What's Happening My First Crisis

Lisa wanted to get off of that subject because she knew that it would only bring stress on Mena, so she changed the subject and asked, "Your first crisis, though? I remember when you were a teenager, you were fourteen years old."

Mena said, "I don't think I know. I found out I had Sickle Cell when I was eleven. My first Sickle Cell Crisis was when we went to Virginia, and I got in that water at the beach in Virginia Beach, and you brought me back. I don't know whose house we were at, but we were at somebody's house, and I was suffering. Did you take me to the hospital? Because I don't remember."

Lisa said, "No, I didn't know what was wrong with you."

Mena lifted her voice and said, "So you let me suffer all night long when you brought me back from Virginia Beach?"

Lisa, in her defense, said, "No, you didn't really say..."

Mena had cut her sentence off and said, "Or did the pain go away?

Lisa said, "It went away, and so you were fine, but then all of a sudden it happened again. Then I went Wow, something is not right with this child and then we took you to our hospital. I remember taking you there, and they said, "You had Sickle Cell." "That's how you ended up going to Johns Hopkins, and then they diagnosed you with HbSC. So, I assumed they didn't know what to do with you."

Mena replied, "Of course they didn't."

Sadly, Lisa said, "See, I remembered that, and when they told me, I just cried."

Mena said, "This is what the Hemoglobin C looks like on her cell phone. Where the arrows are pointing, you see how they are messed up."

Lisa replied, "Ya'll, they are."

Mena went on to say, "So, I had a whole bunch of red blood cells mess up all in my body at one time."

Lisa said, "They almost look like they are half and half."

Mena observes the cells closer, "Yeah, they do, but it's probably from the cells bursting and dying. It's probably from where you know your red blood cells that they die after a while."

Lisa said, "So give me one story that you think."

Mena interrupted Lisa again, "Oh, one more thing. The Hemoglobin Sickle C Disease can develop mild um, chronic hemolysis, causing destruction of your red blood cells. The red blood cells are destroyed prematurely. The body cells can't replace them. So, Splenomegaly is an enlarged spleen. The crescent moon red blood cells get stuck in the spleen's blood vessels, blocking the flow and causes the spleen to enlarge. In other words your blood vessels become blocked by the sickled cells which causes blood pooling and enlargement of the spleen. Your spleen can become ruptured which is life threatening and jaundice occurs. That's another type of difference. Um, a lot of people who have SS usually have jaundiced-looking eyes. Um, which is because the liver is working overtime. You know your liver is like a filter."

They both said it at the same time. Lisa knew that because her uncle had liver disease.

Mena continued on.

"So, it's trying to filter out, but it can't filter because it's over, it's overwhelmed."

Lisa began to think about Mena's side, where she was having so much pain, so she asked Mena the question, "What's happening to your side?"

Mena answered Lisa and said, "They do not know yet."

Lisa said, "That's where you seem to be having so much pain."

Mena said, "And it's up under my rib cage, which they're thinking is my liver. When I lived in Texas, that's where I got my gallbladder taken out. My liver enzymes weren't right. I wonder if they have checked my liver enzymes while I'm here. I'm going to have them do that."

Eyeballs

Lisa once again wanted to make sure that she was getting all this right. Mena had given her so much information that was overwhelming.

Lisa said, "So, for some patients who have HbSC, some doctors will call it Sickle Cell Hemoglobin C disease . What's the worst thing about it besides the pain? Like, what does it do as far as affecting your life?"

Mena replied, "It affects my eyes, which is a big thing for me, especially because I have a fear of eyeballs."

Lisa said, "Eyeballs."

Mena said, "Yes."

Lisa asked and laughed at the same time, "When did you have a fear of eyeballs?"

Mena said, "It's disgusting. They are squishy, they look weird, and they have a long optical cord hanging from the base. It's just disgusting. If anything, ugh."

Mena felt as though she was ready to vomit. Lisa said, "Oh gosh, don't even think about it if it's making you sick. That's terrible."

Mena said, "I can't. I can deal with anything else but that. Amelia and them be teasing me, I can't take it."

Lisa replied, "You've got big eyeballs," and then laughed some more.

Mena said, "Yes, which I don't like looking at sometimes. Like my eyes are different, but when my kids get something they..."

Time To Go Home

Lisa finally interrupted Mena and said, "I gotta go."

Mena said, without getting mad, "Well, we can continue our mommy-daughter talk later."

Lisa said, "Well, the next time we talk, I want to know about family, like how it has affected your life itself. Everybody knows you have pain and how it has affected you physically, but I want to know what your life is like, how it has affected you as a person, as a mother."

Mena said, "Well, it affects, that's a lot."

Lisa said, "I know that's why I said we will do it some other time. I want to hear some stories about how it has interfered with your life."

Mena said, "Well, working is one of them.

Lisa said, "I want to know how it has affected your relationship with friends and your children."

Mena continued, "I have surprisingly good friends who support me all the time. I'm not going to say fairly good friends. I have great friends who check on me, make sure I am alright. If I wasn't all right, they'd come down here and take me where I need to go."

Lisa went on to say, "Do you feel like it has affected your relationship with them sometimes?" Mena said, "No."

Lisa said, "You know, like your demeanor."

Mena said, "NOPE."

Lisa knew that statement wasn't true because she had spoken with a few of Mena's friends, and they all said it was terribly hard to deal with Mena when she was in pain. She didn't always say pleasant things to them. In fact, there were times when their friendship was strained and never fully repaired. However, her true friends have continued to stick around through thick and thin.

Lisa really had to go, so she said, "Alright, we will talk about it another time. I really have to go."

Lisa left happy and satisfied, because for the first time on her visit with her daughter, they didn't argue or disagree on anything. The key was patience. Lisa had really listened to her daughter without interruptions. Lisa remembered that the tortoise turtle was very patient in getting to where it wanted to go. That's why it is so intelligent. A tortoise is able to look at and learn about its surroundings. Lisa had learned so much about her daughter's condition in one visit to the hospital as in all the years that she had let go by. She was truly taking in knowledge about her daughter's condition. She let Mena say all the things she wanted to say. She didn't hear those words coming from her daughter's mouth, "Nobody's Listening."

Lisa smiled to herself as she left. It had taken years–and one long, slow visit–but she'd finally gotten through her daughter's shell—a shell she had created around her for protection. Just like the tortoise, all it took was time.

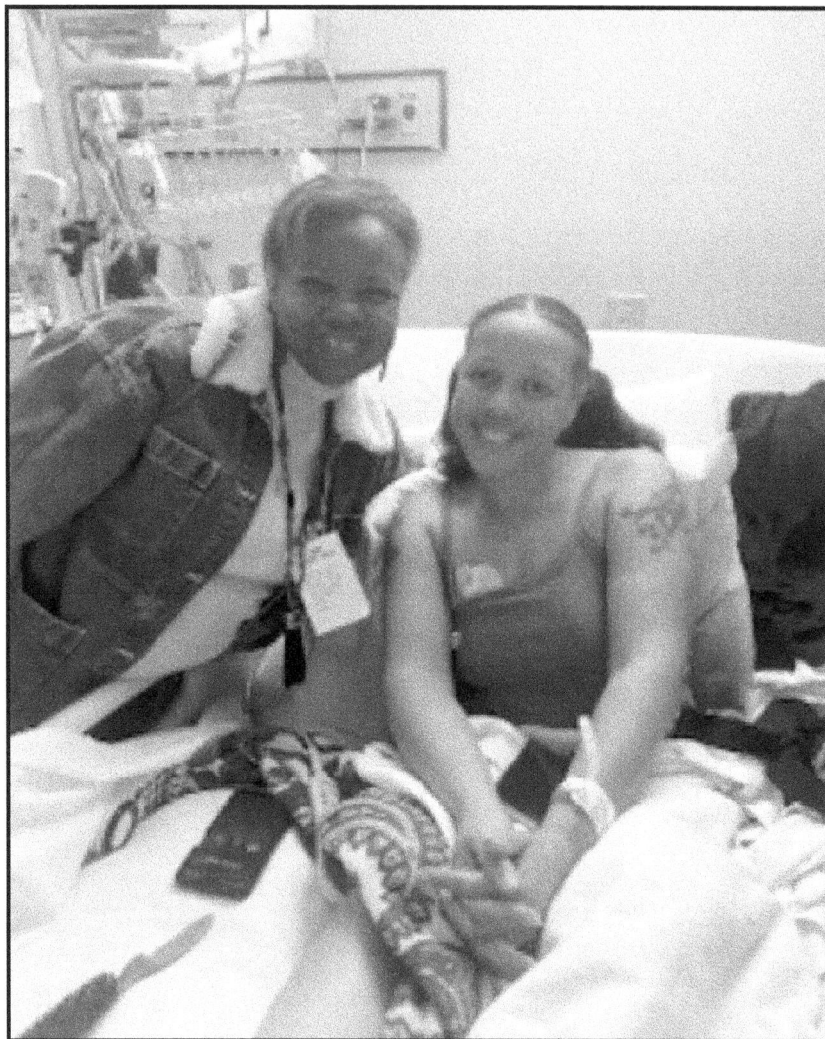

Chapter 23

Sickle Cell Awareness Month (Blue Skies)

Blue Skies is creative or visionary and unconstrained by practicalities. (Blue skies in slang: a time or situation marked by easy progress or success. Growth is back to its old powerhouse levels; there seems to be nothing but blue sky ahead on the inflation front.) Amity Shlaes https://merriam-webster.com

Before such blue skies actually arrive, however, several major problems will have to be resolved. Harry F. Walters et al.

Any opinions expressed in the examples do not represent those of Merriam-Webster or its editors.

Awareness Month Packets For Schools

Sickle Cell Awareness Month usually takes place in September. They talk about living everyday life with Sickle Cell. Mena is a strong warrior, but a mother first. Mena is admired for her strength and endurance, as well as being an advocate for others. She is very into supporting the fundraiser for Sickle Cell Warriors.

"If you've ever had a problem with the doctors at the hospital, let me know," Mena was trying to get a case together. They need to treat ones with Sickle Cell accordingly. Not everyone is the same. Mena was always fighting for herself and others. "If you've ever had a problem, you need to be more knowledgeable about several types of Sickle Cell and what needs to be done to get the pain under control. Because of them, I cannot make any place my home. I am hoping I can lead the way for future leaders regarding Sickle Cell.

Mena began to relate an incident that happened to her at the hospital. "I have had heart palpitations and pain. Should I go to the ER? I'm scared to go to sleep without adult supervision. I went to the hospital, and they sent me home. I am still having palpitations and pain. The hospital is horrible. So, I am waiting to go back to Virginia."

Mena thought about a film she believed all doctors should watch. "In Sickness and in Health" illustrates the emotional toll of illness and the profound love required to care for someone over the long term. She hoped it would open their hearts to what people with Sickle Cell disease go through every day. She especially likes the subtitle "Can True Love Heal All."

Mena wondered where she should begin with advocating for those with Sickle Cell. In deep thought, she said, "I will put a PowerPoint together with the help of my mom to educate children on Sickle Cell. We will start with my kids first and ask every school for permission to educate them. Coloring books will be supplied for the younger ones and self-care packets for the older ones."

Unaware of Mena, her mother was right on it. Lisa had asked the principal where she worked if she could put packets together and hand them out at the PTA meeting for their school. Lisa had also put together a survey to gauge the community's knowledge about Sickle Cell. The outcome was beyond what her heart could bear. 70% of the survey respondents knew absolutely nothing about how you get Sickle Cell. To Lisa's surprise, they didn't even know whether they were born with it or not. Approximately 85% of the families didn't know if they had been tested for Sickle Cell Disease. 90% of the families didn't know which parent had the Sickle Cell Trait, including Lisa. Lisa also had pictures and information about Sickle Cell Disease to educate anyone who would listen or offer a helping hand in spreading the information to the public, whether through typed information or a website to visit. It was information for all races, cultures, and nationalities.

A Change In the School System

Lisa knew that she would have to start small, right in her community, collecting Data to help those with Sickle Cell Disorders. Lisa was so grateful to have parents who were helping in this mission. The school had certain days when you could wear jeans by supporting an organization to raise money. Lisa inquired about it and sent an email to the Board of Directors because the local schools were not in charge of that. The Board of Directors responded and said that they couldn't put it on the calendar for the year because the budgets and schedules were already set for the year. Lisa asked the school if she could try to sell flowers at an event where they were trying to raise money for those who needed to travel to another hospital outside the area. Lisa's request was granted, and they did pretty well with the fundraiser. In the following years, the PTA was no longer at their school due to a loss of interest and a lack of parents taking the lead in volunteering to become part of the PTA board. The change of the principal and Vice principal stops their mission in its tracks. Soon, everything that they had accomplished got lost by the wayside. Lisa still has the information and prizes swiped away in her garage. Lisa knew that someday she would gain the strength to kindle the fire in her heart to start the fight again. If it weren't going to be her, she knew it would be her daughter. Sure enough, her daughter is a Sickle Cell Warrior fighting for those in her community.

Finally, A Basis For Hope

Lisa thought and envisioned nothing but "Blue Skies." Things would start going well for their efforts, and there would be a promising future for those who have Sickle Cell. Lisa didn't believe in luck, but she believed in prayer. Today may not be the day, or even tomorrow, but the future of fighting this battle for a cure will become a reality. Lisa has already seen a change in the school system where she lives. All staff are required to take Safe Schools, and part of it includes a section on Sickle Cell, followed by a small quiz at the end. It identifies everyone's role in learning about Sickle Cell and what to do about it. All staff are required to pass this section online. Lisa knew that she would provide as much support as possible. Some things she would support, and some things she couldn't. Her belief in the matter of blood was blocking the way for her to move in the direction her daughter had moved. They had differences about the use of blood. They both hope that the use of blood will not be the answer to solve the problem for those with Sickle Cell Anemia. Taking blood only treats the disorder temporarily; it's not a cure for this disease. Mena spoke to her daughter, Ivy, who worked in the medical field, and she advised her that it wasn't in her best interests to undergo many blood transfusions. Mena was looking for those blue skies that symbolize trust, loyalty, wisdom, confidence, intelligence, faith, truth, and heaven.

Blue Sky Feeling

Mena thought about waking up all those who had been sleeping for generations, hoping that others would listen and pay attention to all the things she had to say. Especially African Americans. It was a shame that so many of her brothers and sisters had been in the darkness, not experiencing the light about what had caused death to come down on so many of them. Having just an ounce of knowledge about Sickle Cell could bring peace and a sense of calmness to a generation that has suffered for so long. The feeling of blue needed to be turned around to the feeling of tranquility. What an impression that could be if only both of them could just master this task at hand. Lisa looked up at the sky. She saw the clouds moving quickly. As Lisa looked at the clouds, they were rushing about. Lisa hated dealing with the conflicts that she had to endure throughout this ordeal. She wanted to be joyous and comfortable in all situations. She didn't want people to be happy about her lack of knowledge, so details about Sickle Cell were particularly important, and she wasn't about to slow down, just like the clouds. She was going to visit as many schools and facilities as possible to spread information about Sickle Cell. Mena and Lisa were not going to let people feel comfortable. *"Blue skies may not come today,"* Lisa thought, *"but Mena and I will keep pushing until they do."* Mena and Lisa were very optimistic about the future. They were relying on their hope. They were determined to overcome all the challenges and adversities that came their way. They held onto hope in their hearts that an innovative solution to the problems would emerge in the near future.

Chapter 24

Breaking News (Guinea Pig)

Guinea Pig may be associated with the fact that English navigators, when returning from South America transporting these animals, frequently stopped in Guinea. The moniker could also have originated from a mispronounced form of the word "Guiana," the name of the region where some guinea pigs were collected. "Britannica," some say that the term "guinea pig," meaning "one subjected to an experiment," was first used in the 1920's. And this expression is still very common today. If someone calls me a "guinea pig," it means that new ideas or methods are tested on me. Https://learningenglish.voanews.com

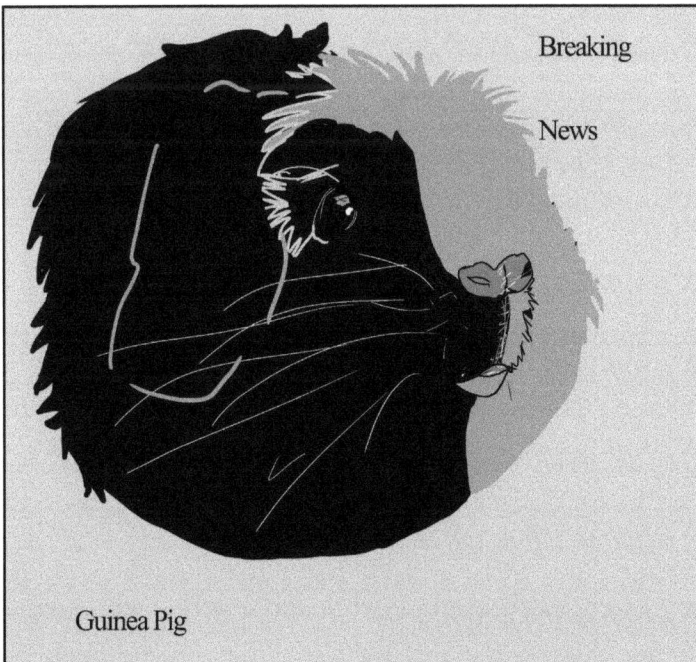

Breaking

News

Guinea Pig

Phone Calls And The News

Now, returning to the phone call between Mena and Lisa, Lisa informed Mena about what she had seen and heard. "Mena, there are a lot of people texting and calling me about the FDA approving First Gene Therapies to Treat Patients with Sickle Cell Disease. I googled it and it said, "Today, the U.S. Food and Drug Administration approved two milestone treatments, Casgevy and Lyfgenia, representing the first cell-based gene therapies for the treatment of Sickle Cell Disease (SCD) in patients 12 years and older. Additionally, one of these therapies, Casgevy, is the first FDA-approved treatment to utilize a type of novel genome editing technology, signaling an innovative advancement in the field of gene therapy."

Mena replied, "Yes, I have been getting a lot of phone calls and texts about it as well. I am excited about it, but I'm not sure if it will be for me or not. I have to read up more on it."

Lisa said, "Well, I am going to send you a link that someone sent me. It was breaking news at 10:00 local news on WSOC. I am going to send you the link wsoctv.com."

Mena listened to the video. Liz Foster said, "Imagine a pain worse than a root canal or a knife twisting in your bone that doesn't go away, that gives you an idea of the pain that comes with Sickle Cell Disease. The disorder causes blood cells to have an abnormal shape that blocks blood flow. Now, Anchor Erica Bryant tells us that Local Physicians at Atrium Health are working on a breakthrough treatment for Sickle Cell Disease."

Enjoli Pettice describes life with Sickle Cell Disease, "it's excruciating pain, you have that feeling of little, tiny people in there on your bones with Jackhammers and then they jackhammer, and they stop and then they jackhammer, and they stop."

"Approximately, one out of 100,000 Americans suffers from chronic illness. For years, doctors have used narcotics or opioids to give patients relief, but the risk of addiction and side effects of withdrawal can lead to more pain. Now, researchers at Atrium Health are studying a new option. I am a firm believer in thinking outside the box. We propose old drugs for new reasons. Dr. IFY OSUNKWO has seen positive results with Suboxone. A medication that has been used to help heroin addicts break free from addiction. Some people think about Suboxone as a medicine to wean you off of hydro narcotics. It actually is a pain medication. It just works in a little bit of a unique way."

Enjoli went on to say, "The new medication in her eyes is a miracle."

The news reporter, Erica Bryant, said, "It changed everything for Enjoli Pettice."

Enjoli said, "Two years ago, I literally was walking with a walker or had to have the use of a cane."

Erica Bryant said, "Now she's gone from needing hospital visits nearly every month to only twice a year."

Enjoli said, "It's miraculous to me to be in the health that I am in now and looking at my future and not worried that Sickle Cell will get in the way."

Liz Foster ended with "In Charlotte, Erica Bryant, Channel 9 Eyewitness News."

Liz Foster reported: "So far, Dr. IFY Osunkwo and her colleagues have seen positive outcomes with about 50 patients. September is Sickle Cell Awareness Month. They plan to publish a finding in a medical journal to help raise awareness about the disease."

Addiction

Mena enjoyed the video, but in her head, she told Lisa, "I remembered that the treatment for the stem cell was costly. I wonder how much this treatment would cost. I had heard about Suboxone, a medication that had been used to help heroin addicts break free from addiction. The generic name for it was buprenorphine. It weans people off of narcotics. Some said that it was highly effective. When I lived in South Carolina, I was taking OxyContin with a higher risk of abuse and Oxycodone lower risk of abuse, and I had to be weaned off them both. Eventually, they would have killed me if I kept taking them for an extended period of time or I would have risked addiction if I kept taking them in high doses."

Lisa asked, "What's the difference between them?"

Mena said, "OxyContin is a time-release that slowly resolves in your body over a course of 12 hours, and Oxycodone extended release takes about 30 to 60 minutes to release in your body. The pain relief lasts for about 4 to 6 hours. One time, a doctor gave me Dilaudid pills 2 milligrams, all within 3 hours, and sent me home. Do you remember when I stayed outside all night long and you couldn't get me back in?"

Lisa, "Yes, I remember, and it was extremely cold outside. No one could make you come back inside. It definitely reminded me of how drug addicts react when they are on drugs. You were rocking back and forth, back and forth, unaware of what was going on around you. In my opinion, so, wonder if those with Sickle Cell get a bad rap that they are drug seeking. It's some of the doctors who don't know much about Sickle Cell or how to treat it, and they overdose on you guys. They send you home too soon to see how the medicines that they give you would react. I'm sure everybody is different."

Lisa was thinking about Mena when she was behaving like someone who had overdosed on drugs.

"That night, I should have called the ambulance, I suppose, but we were thinking this too would pass. We were thinking that you would just pull out of it, as you always have. I sent the kids to bed so that they wouldn't see you like that. I just told them you're going to be alright. You'll see them in the morning. They believed me and went off to bed, deeply saddened. I was so glad when a doctor who knew what he was doing gradually weaned you off of both of the drugs. You were a mess."

Mena said, "You were right about that. I am going to look into this treatment, though, because just to test for the Stem Cell, it costs $500, and one of my closest friends, Michelle, is going to pay for it. I told her no."

Lisa said, "The way that you are in pain, I don't think I could make it. If I knew there was something out there to stop it, I would. If she is offering, let her. I have seen you in pain too often. How in the world could you want to keep going through that?"

Mena said, "I suppose you're right. I'm going to help her at least pay for half of it. I will get right on it. The only thing, Mom, is that you have to go through radiation treatments first. That's what is holding me back. It can kill off all your cells, and that is what makes this treatment so risky."

Lisa said, "Having Sickle Cell is risky as well; it causes death."

Mena said, "I suppose you're right. Eventually, it will kill me, or the damage it causes to my body will kill me. In the meantime, I am going to look into this Gene Therapy too."

The fact remains, Mena didn't want to be anyone's guinea pig. But if this treatment or new idea could offer a real chance of being released from this deadly disease—not just an experiment—she was willing to try.

Chapter 25

I Don't Remember (Elephant)

Elephant—TRUE! Elephants are the largest land mammals on Earth and have a remarkable memory to match their massive size. While the old saying may be exaggerated, it's truer than not. An elephant's memory is key to its survival and, sometimes, its herd's. Herds have a matriarchal structure, with one older female at the head. These dominant females have developed a bank of knowledge over their years that helps them survive in the wild. A matriarch will remember the location of a reliable water source and lead the herd to it. Time and distance don't impact their ability to lead their herd to the right place, demonstrating their superb memory when it comes to their spatial environment. Evidence of their great memories is also seen in social behavior. When confronted with an unfamiliar elephant, matriarchs will assume defensive positions toward it because they realize that these animals could pose a threat. When they come across an elephant that they have interacted with before, even if it was many years ago, they become very animated and excited to be reunited. Elephants use their 10.5-pound brains to encode necessary identification and survival information to keep their herd safe in the wild. https://www.clevelandzoosociety.org

Matriarch Of The Family

Have you ever heard the saying "An elephant never forgets?" Mena had failed to remember so many things. She either had put some things out of her mind or had neglected to do things. There were times when Mena seemed to be in a black hole where nothing seemed to be centered around her. She was oblivious to who or what was around her. Mena would also fail to remember or recall things she had said or done. Mena was not one to overlook any situation. She was always on top of things. It was as if she had amnesia, total or partial memory loss about any situation that had taken place or something that had happened years ago. Remembering these things was what made Mena the matriarch, just like the elephant of the family. She was the matriarch of the family because a male in her life was not currently in the plans. She had become a very independent woman. She had set in her mind that she wasn't going to be controlled by others or influenced by others. She was doing fine by herself. All her thinking and the way she acted was her prerogative. Mena said to herself that she was not subject to anyone's authority, especially when it came to the doctors who thought they knew what she wanted or needed. Their words seemed to find themselves thrown right out of the window.

When Mena was admitted to the hospital, she was still trying to give out orders to her household as to what to do and what not to do. She had lost her ability to be the matriarch of the family. Mario and Amelia had to take control of the family.

It wasn't until Lisa, their grandmother, threatened them with her words, "I'll be over this afternoon, and the house better be cleaned or you're not going anywhere."

Lisa didn't dare to tell Mena that there were times when they didn't follow her directions for fear of adding stress to Mena, which would cause her more pain all over her body. The kids continued to eat when they wanted, and not only that, but they also ate what they wanted. When Mena would send money for them to go grocery shopping, they bought what they wanted. Eating healthy foods was no longer on their list. They had decided to take advantage of every situation they possibly could while Mena was dealing with her Sickle Cell Crisis at the hospital.

Mena's Defensive Protection

When Mena was at home, just like an elephant's social life, Menu would assume defensive protection with her family's social interaction with others. Mena never let strangers come into her home, not even answering the door if she didn't know who they were. One time, a census lady came to the door to stress the importance of filling out a form about her household so that the schools and neighborhood would benefit from it. Mena didn't care about her; she was a stranger and a bother. A politician came by so that she could get her vote. It was as if she was a threat to her family. Mena completely ignored her knocks at the door. The kids looked out the window and watched her walk away. No one was going to invade her family space or living quarters. Anyone walking past her house posed a threat, especially if it was a man. Instead of her protecting the kids, they were protecting her. It took Mena 5 years to let her guard down to even communicate with her neighbor. However, there were times, just like elephants that had interacted with other elephants a long time ago, when they were excited to be united again. Mena was the same way: if someone came to the door and she hadn't seen them for twenty years or so, she would remember and perk right up with the biggest smile and laughter. Mena had acquired a lot of knowledge about life in general over the years. She had lived in the countryside, suburbs, and cities. The city taught Mena how to fight, protect herself, manage her household affairs, and avoid being taken advantage of, sometimes for the better and sometimes not for the best. Elephants use necessary identification and survival information to lead their families. Mena knew where all the reliable resources were to meet her own needs and those of her family for survival. The thrift stores, Homeless shelters, Food Banks, Free Healthcare Facilities, and, yes, Child Support from their fathers.

Missing In Action

The loss of Mena's memory and her being sick were overwhelming. She had missed so much of her life not being a part of it.

"Mena, do you remember when we had a family reunion? Oh yeah, you weren't there."

"Mena, do you remember what happened at the family picnic? Oh yeah, you weren't there."

"Mena, do you remember what happened at the funeral? Oh yeah, you weren't there."

"Mena, do you remember what a fun time we had when we were on vacation? "Oh yeah, you weren't there."

"Mena, do you remember your doctor's appointment? Oh yeah, that's right, you weren't there."

"Mena, do remember when you were mean and cruel to me, and I didn't deserve it. "Oh yes, you weren't there to remember."

Time began to interfere with Mena's memory. Some days she couldn't remember what day of the week it was. Often, she would think it was morning when it was nighttime. She didn't know if the sun was shining or whether it was a cloudy, rainy day, especially at the hospital where there were no windows. Holidays and Birthdays often went by the wayside. It seemed as if she was often sick around the same time every year when it came to major holidays. At Christmas and Thanksgiving, she didn't remember anything about those special days, so she didn't bother to celebrate them the way others did or spend time with any of her close family, except for her children. Mena had missed uniting with her family and friends often because of her pain and the drugs the doctors had prescribed for her to take. The medicines were just swiping out her memory of so many things.

When pictures were being taken at the family reunion with her family, uncles, aunts, and cousins, she was missing in action. It affected her so much that her children also stopped attending special gatherings. They had begun to feel like strangers to everyone, even though their outside families surrounded them. Lisa once remembered when her mother's side of the family was having a family reunion, and her grandchildren, Mario and Amelia, had disappeared. She found them sitting in a truck.

Lisa approached them and said, "Why are you guys sitting in the truck?"

Mario said, "Because in the house, while we were sitting, they said, 'Who are you? They acted as if we didn't belong there, so we left.'"

Amelia said, "Yep, and we are not going back. We will sit here and wait for you."

Lisa knew at the moment they meant it, and her family reunion would be cut short. They were just like their Mother, Mena, defensive around anyone they didn't know, family or not. Lisa knew the family just wanted to get to know them.

A Mind Is Terrible Thing To Waste

"Yes, a mind is such a terrible thing to waste, but a wonderful thing to invest in." This is the iconic slogan of the United Negro College

Fund (UNCF). It underscores, in a few short words, the life-changing effect of a college education on people of every racial or ethnic origin.

Lisa thought of the first part of it, "A mind is a terrible thing to waste." She thought about the mind. Lisa looked at her phone and googled it. The dictionary definition from Oxford Languages uses the noun- 1. The element of a person that enables them to be aware of the world and their experiences, to think, and to feel, is the faculty of consciousness and thought.

A person's intellect.

A person's memory

A person identified with their intellectual faculties.

A person's attention

Verb-1.be distressed, annoyed, or worried by.

Have an objection to

Be reluctant

Informal

2. Regard as important; feel concerned about.

Used to urge someone to remember or take care to bring about something

Used to warn someone to avoid injury or damage from a hazard.

Phrase

Bear something in mind

Remember a fact or circumstance and take it into account.

"You need to bear in mind that the figures vary from place to place."

Lisa felt that part of Mena was being robbed in so many ways of the ability to feel emotions, the ability to think, and the ability to comprehend things in a timely and rightful manner. The doctors and meds were robbing Mena of who she was and is.

Mena wrote in her journal:

I am illumination. I am the glow that brightens your day. I spent my Born Day in the hospital, but I'm still blessed. Not everyone has made it to 46. Nature is healing. The sun regenerates me, and the moon energizes me. My children are my legacy. I love them because I love me. They are me and I am them.

Chapter 26

Mena (Mother Nature)

Mother Nature- (sometimes known as Mother Earth or the Earth Mother) is a personification of nature that focuses on the life-giving and nurturing aspects of nature by embodying it in the form of a mother or mother goddess. https://en.wikipedia.org

Personality Change

Mena had always dreamed of being a good mother, but sometimes all the things that had been centered around her always seemed to get in her way. Just like Mother Nature, she wanted to provide her children with all the resources that they could possibly need. If it meant being supported by the state, she would accept whatever she could receive. For now, she was receiving disability, and that was a tremendous help, because she was unable to work. She was unable to keep a job because of her Sickle Cell. She was determined that she was going to try to be the best mother figure she possibly could be. She often wondered how others saw her as a mother figure. There were times when she was feeling great with laughter, joy, and a song in her heart. Why couldn't what was troubling her inside just leave her alone? Mena had always thought that she was Bipolar. Her mother, Lisa, had even mentioned it from time to time. Bipolar Disorder created mood swings in Mena. Mena had all the signs of depression and mania. She cried out of nowhere and had elevated, extreme changes in her mood or emotions. Her energy level and her activity level changed often. This affected Mena's mental activity, physical immobility, and behavior. She would often change from being her usual self. It had definitely been noticed by her family and friends. Mena was just like Mother Nature. Her personality was just like the seasons. She was like the warm days of spring. She was like the hot days of Summer and the cold days of winter. Her temperament was like rainy days, sunny days, snowy days, and fall days filled with beauty. Her greatest strength was caring for her children, just like nature that replenishes itself. She was going to pass her roots of life on to her children with mildness, joy, goodness, kindness, and love. Mena's strongest root was not self-control or patience. That was something she was working on. Maybe they would inherit that from their grandmother, Lisa. She was going to be rooted with care and nourishment, even though she knew it would be a struggle for her every day.

80's Party

There were times when Mena couldn't even sleep at night. She would go through these emotional crashes, which left her depressed and worn out. That's why she would have problems getting along with others. There were times when her emotions were dominated by excessive and persistent irritability. Mena often thought about nature helping her out when she was feeling this way. She was especially fond of the moon because that's the time she was most active. It seemed to guide her along the way. The moon's gravity balanced the Earth, which in turn balanced her. Mena had dysphoria. There were times when Mena couldn't move her body or body parts. She felt very unhappy, uneasy with others, or just not satisfied with what others were doing around her. Most of all, she wasn't happy with herself.

Lisa remembered a time when Mena was going to go to a party across the bridge. Mena was so excited. By evening, Mena had changed her mind.

"Mom," Mena shouted, "I'm going to my best friend's '80s party. I was going through some pictures that were taken of me in the '80s. I was looking good. I had long flowing hair, and my body was 26-28-26. I had a flat stomach and firm muscles in my arms and legs.

Lisa said, "Well, I hope you have a great time. You need to get out of this house and enjoy your time of not just thinking about your responsibilities of being a mother."

Mena responded, "You got that right! It's time for me to go out and have some fun."

Putting Mood Swings Under Control

Mena didn't like to leave her children often, because when she was feeling great, she wanted to spend quality time with them. Those days had been spent scarish throughout her life. Mena wanted to nurture her children as other mothers had done. She often thought of her sister, Ivy, who spent a lot of quality time with her kids. Every time she turned around, they were going to recitals, fishing, going to the beach, and traveling together. Mena wanted her days to be spent with her children doing exciting things as well. However, Mena had the temperament of Mother Nature. When she was with them, they were happy sunny days, and then a stormy day could pop up at any moment, where she would yell and scream at them for no reason. Having Sickle Cell was a big part of it.

Mena knew that she had Premenstrual Dysphoric Disorder (PMDD). It was an abnormal reaction to normal hormone changes that happen with each menstrual cycle. The hormone changes can cause a serotonin deficiency. It's a substance found naturally in the brain and intestines that constricts blood vessels and can affect mood, as well as cause physical symptoms. Mena had researched PMDD from a website that said, How does someone get dysphoric disorder? The website was hopkinsmedicine.org. When Mena meditated on the information from this website, she discussed it with her doctor and decided to have a partial hysterectomy to try to solve the problem that she was having every month. What do you know? It did help a lot. She had gone forward with this operation because she didn't want to lose any unnecessary blood if she didn't have to. She also wanted her mood swings to be put under control.

Something Has Gone Wrong

Lisa had returned that evening to see what Mena looked like. She couldn't wait to see what Mena had picked out from the shopping that day. What outfit would she have picked out? Would it be a dress, a jumper, or pants with an elegant top? Would the outfit be red, yellow, or blue? It would probably be blue because that was Mena's favorite color. Oh, and what pair of shoes and accessories would Mena have picked out? Upon entering the house, Lisa removed her shoes and rushed back to Mena's bedroom. Lisa knocked on Mena's door.

Lisa said, "Mena, I'm back."

Mena replied in a frustrated voice, "You should have called me first."

Lisa knew what that meant. It meant Mena's demeanor had changed since this morning. Something had gone wrong. Lisa opened the door to Mena's bedroom.

Mena said, "Yes, Mom, what is it?"

Lisa said, "I thought you were going to the '80s party across the bridge. What happened? Did they cancel it?"

Mena answered and said, "No! I just don't feel like going."

Lisa replied, "Didn't you go shopping for a new outfit?"

Mena replied, "No, Mom. You're always asking me questions. I was looking at my yearbook, and I don't look the same. I was so much prettier than and three sizes smaller. I looked in the mirror and I just looked tired. I decided not to go shopping, so I went into my closet, and nothing could fit me.

Lisa looked at her daughter, trying to think of the right thing to say that wouldn't irritate Mena, as she always seemed to do. Lisa knew that it would be a difficult task, if not impossible, to bring Mena out of this state of mind. She knew that once Mena had gone through something terrifying to her, disheartening, or an intrusive thought, she usually would never snap out of it.

Lisa knew Mena would be yelling, "You don't get it. You just don't understand how I am feeling." She would want to be by herself. Just left alone.

A Breakthrough

Lisa was prepared for what she thought would happen. Lisa said to Mena, "I went through the same thing that you are going through. I didn't want to go to my class reunion either, because I have changed a lot. I had to tell myself to accept the things I could not change. I begin to think about how I could enhance my look. I am a beautiful black woman that God has created. Wine gets better with time, just in a different way. I attended that class reunion, and I received numerous compliments on my dress and appearance. I know that your father and I made beautiful girls who have come into this world. Inside as well as outside. Mena, you and I don't often do things together, but I would like to make this event happen for you."

Lisa knew Mena like a book, so she prepared some things for Mena just in case she didn't follow through with preparing herself for the class reunion. "Look at what I bought for you. Do you like this dress? It's made of satin to enhance those curves of yours, and it has sequins of beads. You will definitely be making a statement as you're dancing on the floor. Your dress will be flowing with elegance. I even bought you the shoes and accessories to match. What do you think? Oh, and you know that I am a makeup artist, so I will apply your makeup. Come on, let's have some fun before you go."

Lisa's heart was racing. She was hoping that she would make a breakthrough in Mena's depression. Hoping her demeanor would change to joy and enlightenment. Yes, happiness.

Mena set her eyes on everything that her mother had done for her, and she said, "Sure, Mom, we can try."

Lisa had made a breakthrough, something that doesn't happen often.

Mena said, "What about the kids?"

Lisa answered, "Oh, they are going to the movies and Planet Maze with me tonight."

Lisa had accomplished a shift in Mena's mood swing. She knew that this would be only temporary, but moments and memories like these were worth all the effort. They would talk about dealing with her mood swings at another time. Lisa also knew that when Mena would return, she would be ready to embrace her children with love. Asking questions like 'Did you enjoy yourself? Did you miss me? I missed you. Are you happy to see me?' I'm glad to be back.

What would you like to do? Should we take a walk in the park, rain or shine? Mena didn't care what the weather forecast would be as long as she and her children could make the best of it. Mother

Nature would always be on her side. Even with the cold weather, she would have to pay the consequences later.

Life-Giving Force

She would be creative just like Mother Nature. Mena knew that it was essential to maintain nature's balance, and the consequences of upsetting it could be severe. She felt the same way about her kids. She had to be balanced in raising and nurturing her children, or there would be severe consequences, with her not being able to deal with raising a family. Just like Nature Mena had acquired a bank of knowledge about how to focus on helping herself first, and then this would help her to be the best mother she could be to help her family. She was going to see her children flourish with time. Mena was going to see to it that her children would be protected, nurtured, and grow with every ounce of power that was left in her.

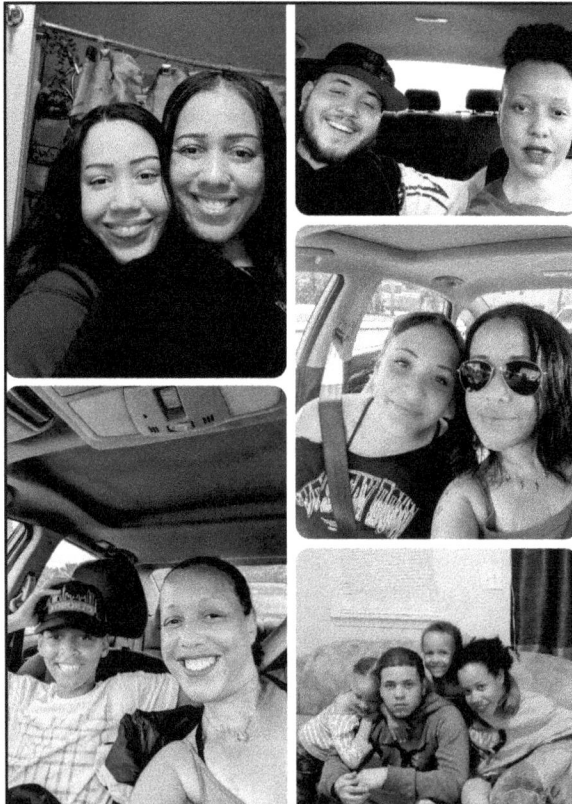

Chapter 27

Happy (Light)

Light is a source of illumination, whether natural (like the sun) or artificial (like your lamp). Light itself, the word can take a lot of different forms. It can be a noun, an adjective, or a verb, and it can mean bright or not heavy. https://vocabulary.com Feeling or showing pleasure or contentment. Satisfaction with a person, arrangement, or situation.

Lisa was visiting Mena's godmother, Bee, under the carport. There was a table with chairs and flowers centered around it. It was used as a gathering place for friends to sit and greet neighbors as they walked by. Mena came running to meet Lisa and Bee. She came to a graceful, slow walk as if she were as light as a feather. The heavy load she always seemed to carry had been put aside for the moment. Mena was so delighted to see Bee. Lisa could see the true meaning of happiness written all over Mena's face when she was embraced by her Bee, whom she hadn't seen in quite some time. Once again, Lisa saw a rare sighting of her daughter. Her physical body and demeanor had no noticeable signs of pain.

Best Friends You Can Count ON

Mena was definitely in a happy frame of mind, a state of satisfaction. She had always loved to see Lisa and Bee together. For she knew they had been best friends since their youth, only to discover that they were cousins. They bonded so well together. She also knew Lisa had several best friends who supported her in her time of need. Mena loved the situation that she was in as well, for she had several best friends and one of them had just recently passed away. She was truly loved by many. Rain had a massive funeral. Almost the whole town was there to say their goodbyes. Mena hopes that if ever she would succumb to this deadly disease that her community would see her as a great advocate, as someone who had shed light on preventive methods for Sickle Cell. She had hoped they too would come and say their goodbyes as well for her. Rain was a strong support for Mena, and Mena for her.

Mena: A Reflection Of Light

The temperament that Lisa often saw in Mena's face was completely gone. At that very moment, Mena was the light of Lisa's Life. Mena's face was so radiant. In the darkness, Lisa could see the reflection of the light shining upon Mena's and Bee's faces as they stood under the light coming from the one Bulb in the carport. Her face had the power of brightness and gleam. Lisa thought to herself, "Have you ever seen the summer night in northern latitudes where the sun barely sets? Any location within the Arctic Circle (or the Antarctic Circle). This truly was a rare moment to see as well. Mena had no coloring on her face because of all the treatments and medicines that she had received to ease her pain and lack of sleep from this deadly disease of Sickle Cell. Mena's skin seemed to get lighter and brighter with time as they stood there. Both Lisa and Bee were so fond of Mena at this moment in every way. Mena was the person they had come to love. Mena was bubbling with happiness and smiling from head to toe. She had that blush of joy that you rarely often would see. Mena had a sparkle in her eye that twinkled like the night stars. She was free from sadness, her troubles, and any weakness that she may have had from this Blood disorder (HbSC) that made Mena weak to her knees. Mena was like the colors of a rainbow. Mena was a reflection of beauty and a symbol of hope to all communities, and especially Sickle Cell Warriors. She was fighting the fine fight with all her might.

Mena glamorized all her pictures from the hospital, especially those with her family, by saying, "Here we go again, but I've got this. Nothing can stop me. Not even myself. About to be set free."

Lisa admired her strength and endurance. Yes, at this moment, Lisa could honestly say to Mena, "I am listening and I C you."

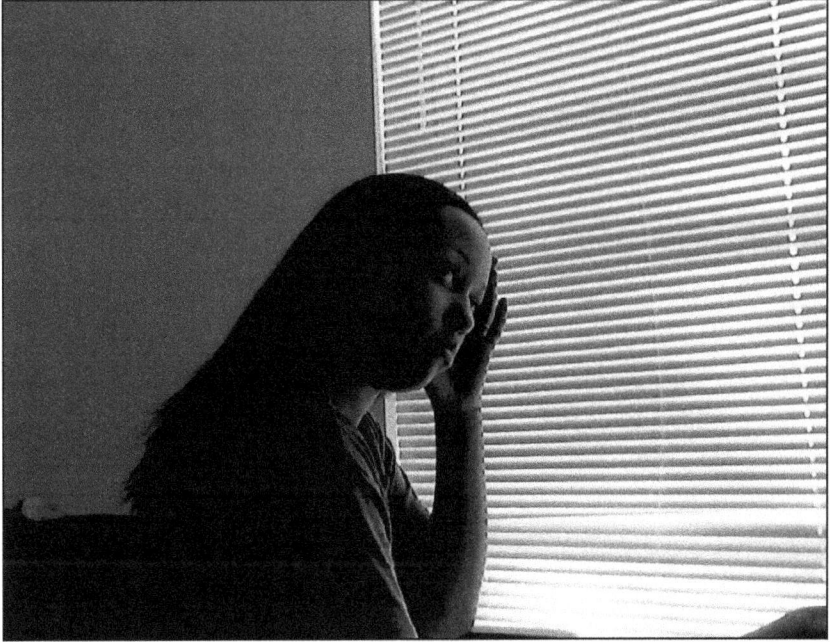

"Open the Blinds and let the light shine."

Afterword

Do you know if you have the Sickle Cell Trait? Most people who have the Sickle Cell Trait are not aware of it, and it puts them at risk of having a child with Sickle Cell Disease; in rare cases, it puts them at risk. Two genes for Sickle Cell Hemoglobin (SS) result in Sickle Cell Anemia, the most severe form of Sickle Cell Disease. In other words, if both a male and female have the Sickle Cell Trait, their children could be at risk of having Sickle Cell Anemia. If you know your hemoglobin status and that of your partner, you'll know if you're likely to have a child with Sickle Cell Disease. Other common forms of Sickle Cell Disease include Sickle Cell Hemoglobin C Disease (SC), Sickle Cell Hemoglobin E Disease (SE), and Sickle Cell Beta Thalassemia Disease (SB). https://ncdhhs.gov

Many of us may be thinking of having children one day, so stop and think very seriously about getting tested. You want to find out if you are a carrier of Sickle Cell Trait. It means your child's life. Hb SS, Hb SC, and Hb S beta thalassemia all these hemoglobin types cause a Vaso-occlusive crisis. With all this said, my husband and I neglected to find out because we didn't know any better. There is now so much information available about Sickle Cell that there is no excuse not to take precautions. It's like saying I didn't know how to protect myself from getting pregnant or from contracting AIDS. It's like putting an umbrella up after it rains. There are so many avenues for getting this information. The internet, television programs, books, word of mouth, videos, stories, pamphlets, seminars, fundraisers, clinics, and sometimes word of mouth.

FOOD FOR THOUGHT FOR DOCTORS

What is the definition of a doctor? A person skilled or specializing in healing arts.

1. Doctored, doctoring

- To give medical treatment

- To restore to good condition

- To adapt or modify for a desired end by alteration or special treatment

2. To alter deceptively (to deprive of genuineness, naturalness, or simplicity).

https://www.merrian-webster.com

Remember why you became a doctor: to take care of people, both mentally and physically. To care for them like you would your family.

Acts 20:35 I have shown you in all things that by working hard in this way, you must assist those who are weak and must keep in mind the words of the Lord Jesus, when he himself said: "There is more happiness in giving than there is in receiving."

Don't forget the giving of your heart along the way.

Listen and truly see your patient.

References

Chapter 1 What's Happening To Me? (Venomous Snake)

Complications of Sickle Cell Disease

People with <u>sickle cell disease</u> (SCD) can experience many complications of the disease. Complications are different for each person and can range from mild to severe. Complications tend to worsen over time.

<u>Symptoms What Are Complications of Sickle Cell Disease?</u>

<u>sickle-cell.com</u>

Chapter 2 The Ride To The Hospital (Waves Of The Sea)

History of Sickle Cell

This article helps families to have an understanding of the background of sickle cell and to have meaningful conversations about sickle cell awareness.

<u>History and Evolution of Sickle Cell Disease</u>

<u>https://www.sparksicklecellchange.com</u>

Chapter 3 Beyond The Pain Of Sickle Cell (Child Birth

<u>What to Know When Planning to Have a Baby | Sickle-Cell.com</u>

When deciding to have a baby this article explains how to make a plan for what to expect. It relates to whether or not you can have a baby with or without risk. It gives you resources to go to for assistance.

Chapter 4 Desensitized (Siblings)

Mental And Health Awareness

This article gears toward counseling and support group resources. Mental health is very critical for everyone's well being. Ex[lore the Therapy Toolkit for Mental Health and Wellness.

Mental Health and Wellness - Sickle Cell Disease Association of America Inc.

Sicklecelldisease.org

Chapter 5 The Dark Room (Moon Flower)

A parents Guide To Managing Sickle Cell

Download information about sickle cell. It's a Parents guide on how to acquire knowledge on how to manage and live with Sickle Cell.

A Parent's Guide to Managing Sickle Cell Disease » Sickle Cell Society

Chapter 6 I Want To Go Home (Monarch Butterfly)

Opioid Overdose in Patients with Sickle Cell Disease, Outcomes Among Hospitalized Patients in the United States: A Nationwide Analysis

Communities struggle with the devastating opioid crisis. In this article it will discuss and analyze the outcome for patient's hospitalization with opioid overdose and how to address concerns that providers have when prescribing opioids to their patients. Opioids are commonly used to manage treatments.

Opioid Overdose in Patients with Sickle Cell Disease, Outcomes Among Hospitalized Patients in the United States: A Nationwide Analysis | Blood | American Society of Hematology

https://doi.org/10.1182/blood-2024-199914

Chapter 7 Moving (Wild Sunflower)

Implications of climatic change on sickle cell anemia: A review

Climate change has emerged as a significant global challenge, influencing environmental conditions worldwide which have a profound effect on sickle cell patients. Explores how climatic variations affect those with Sickle Cell. Topic discussed will be prevalence, management, and outcomes of SCA. Discussions on weather patterns, temperature, increased frequency of extreme weather events, and variations in humidity levels will be addressed.

Implications of climatic change on sickle cell anemia: A review - PMC

Chapter 8 Sickle Cell Trait or Sickle Cell Disease Diagnosis (Marsh Marigold or Celandine)

Difference between a flower and a weed-

It's your perception in the way you view them. It's a very informative article to explain the difference.

https://sciencing.com

by Meg Michelle updated March 24,2022

Sickle Cell Trait vs. Sickle Cell Disease

Read to find out the difference between Sickle Cell Trait and Sickle Cell Disease. It speaks of the risk of complications and the severity.

Sickle Cell Trait vs. Sickle Cell Disease | Pfizer

https://www.pfizer.com

Chapter 9 Inherited Trait (Cry Wolf)

Living Well- Managing Stress, Sleep and Dreaming, Understanding emotions

Our content helps you make the best choices for your mental well-being: Meditation, Therapy, Relationships, Self-Improvement, Depression, Anxiety

Our team of board-certified physicians and other mental health professionals ensures our content is accurate, up-to-date, and inclusive. https://www.verywellmind.com

Verywell Mind's content is for informational and educational purposes only. Our website is not intended to be a substitute for professional medical advice, diagnosis, or treatment.

Chapter 10 We Have To Let You Go (Autumn Leaf)

Root rot and fungal infections- https://www.urbanmali.com

A challenging aspect of living with sickle cell disease (SCD) can be finding and keeping a job. This article explores some of these challenges and how to overcome them.

Sickle Cell and Employment - A Guide for Employers and Employees on Work, Employment and Sickle Cell Disorder (SCD) http://sicklecellwork.dmu.ac.uk

Chapter 11 Journal Writing (Fossils)

Mayo Clinic speaks on topics as to why hydroxyurea is used on cancer patients as well as sickle cell patients. Speaks on the side effects, how it may lessen the pain in sickle cell patients episodes, different dosage forms, side effects, dangers, proper use and solution.

Hydroxyurea (oral route) - Side effects & dosage - Mayo Clinic
March 01, 2025

https://www.mayoclinic.org

Chapter 12 Relationships (Love Birds)

Living with Sickle Cell Disease -SHANIQUA'S SICKLE CHONICLES

How To Maintain A Healthy Relationship With Sickle Cell

Topic on how you can navigate being overly tired, making a care plan, pain management, and more. She speaks on how Sickle Cell can impact your relationships that go beyond physical systems. How it can put a strain on your partner and the connection of bonding together.

How to maintain a healthy romantic relationship with sickle cell disease Feb 14,2025

https://sicklecellanemianews.com

Recommended Reading- Here's What I've Learned About Dating With Sickle Cell Disease February 5, 2021

Chapter 13 Hands Up (Spider Lily)

The Red Spider Lily And Why Its Name Is Synonymous With Death (defendersblog.org)

The Red Spider Lily And Why Its Name Is Synonymous With Death - defendersblog

https://defendersblog.org

Golden lily or yellow spider- Content Hub | UC Agriculture and Natural Resources Sept 25,2020

https://ucanr.edu

Search American Addiction Centers

American Addiction Centers Topics-OxyContin vs. Oxycodone: Differences and Similarities (Aug 23,2024), Side Affects and Dangers of Misuse (Jul 19,2024, and Oxycodone Withdrawal Symptoms, Timeline and Detox Treatment (May 16,2025)

Chapter 14 Rare Sighting (Two Moons)

Sickle Cell Complications-Supporting Patients with SCD. Every patient is affected by SCD differently, Dactylitis (Hand-Foot Syndrome) Painful swelling in the hands and feet is usually the first symptom of SCD in infants and toddlers. It is caused by sickled cells getting stuck in the blood vessels and blocking blood flow in the small bones of hands and feet. This often happens in adults as well. **https://www.cdc.gov**

How do you treat a swollen hand with sickle cell? Treatment also usually involves bed rest, immobilization, and use of a hot pack to ease discomfort and swelling. People should avoid cold packs because severe colds can tighten blood vessels and reduce blood flow. Episodes of dactylitis may be triggered by: Cold exposure, Dehydration, Infection, and Injury. Extreme pain with fever, fluids given by IV may be necessary. Antibiotics may treat or prevent infections that could trigger dactylitis. **https://sickle-cell.com**

Chapter 15 Mena's Waking Moments And Sleepless Nights (Different Phases Of The Moon)

Full Moon-https://Moongiant.com

(Moon Phase Explained Animations and Time-lapse) https://m.youtube.com

Exploring the relationship of sleep, cognition, and cortisol in Sickle Cell disease

People with SCD took longer to fall asleep, had greater wake bouts, mobile minutes, and fragmented sleep. People with SCD experienced a flattened diurnal cortisol profile. Sleep disturbances might interfere with diurnal cortisol rhythm and contribute to lower cognitive scores. **https://www.sciencedirect.com**

Sleep Disturbance in Adults with Sickle Cell Disease: Relationships with Executive and Psychological Functioning - PMC

Chapter 16 The Next Visit (Salmon and Fiddler Crabs)

The article gives tips on traveling. The complications of traveling. Are there risks with traveling?

What Are Tips for Traveling by Airplane with Sickle Cell Disease?

sickle-cell.com

Places to live if you have Sickle Cell- <u>inspire.com</u>

<u>Best cities a cross the world to live with sickle cell SC disease - Sickle cell anemia</u>

Chapter 17 I'm Free (Briar)

National Library of Medicine (National Center for Biotechnology Information

Use of infusion ports in patients with sickle cell disease: Indications and complications. Information will describe why this procedure is necessary for some sickle cell patients. Abstract: Background, Methods, Results and Conclusion

<u>Use of infusion ports in patients with sickle cell disease: Indications and complications - PubMed</u> Copyright 2021 Wiley Periodicals LLC

pubmed.ncbi.nlm.nih.gov

Chapter 18 Rainy Days And Mondays Always Get Me Down (Rhododendrons)

Red Cell Exchange in Sickle Cell Disease

Topics discussed are red cell exchange transfusion, sickle cell anemia, hemoglobin, transfusion, exchange transfusion, whole blood, viscosity, oxygen, blood viscosity

<u>Red Cell Exchange in Sickle Cell Disease | Hematology, ASH Education Program | American Society of Hematology</u>

<u>https://doi.org/10.</u>

Chapter 19 Everything Coming At Me From Different Directions (Snowflakes)

What's Your Story?

Depression, Anxiety, and Sickle Cell Disease

Reviewed by: HU Medical Review Board/ Last reviewed: January 2-21/ Last updated: December 2020

Topics: What is anxiety? Why does sickle cell disease cause depression and anxiety? How does mental health affect individuals' outcomes? What are treatment options? <u>Depression, Anxiety, and Sickle Cell Disease</u>

<u>Sickle-cell.com</u>

Chapter 20 People Are Staying Here Too Long (Animal Control)

Rights For Sickle Cell Patients

Sickle Cell patients are protected under certain federal laws and advocacy efforts such as: Public education, Medicaid and other health programs.

<u>Sickle Cell Disease Fact</u>

SCDAA Statement: Know Your Rights In The Emergency Department June 20,2024

This article speaks of Medicare & Medicaid promoting new resources. It gives reminders of knowing your rights in the emergency room. A reference is under the Emergency Medical Treatment and Labor Act, it is known as EMTALA.

<u>SCDAA Statement: Know Your Rights in the ER - Sickle Cell Disease Association of America Inc.</u>

<u>sicklecelldisease.org</u>

The Checkup by Single Care

THE CHECKOUT

How to refuse to fill a prescription tactfully

Pharmacists sometimes have to decline an Rx. Here's how to do it with the least amount of upset. By Gerardo Sison, Pharm.D./Apr.7,2022

This article mentions Key takeaways: Pharmacists can refuse to fill a prescription for several reasons such as potential abuse or misuse, ordering the prescription to be refilled too soon, personal or religious beliefs, or it may not be within the state laws and company policies.

When can a pharmacist refuse to fill a prescription?

https://www.singlecare.com

Home - Health Services Cost Review Commission (HSCRC)

Hospital rate regulation in Maryland was established by an act of the Maryland legislature in 1971. The law created the Health Services Cost Review Commission (HSCRC), an independent State agency with seven Commissioners

Chapter 21 Misfit (Shrub Rose)

The burdens of SCD on patients

There are times when SCD patients have burdens in their lives. The article explains the psychological, physical, and social effects that causes a toll on patients with sickle cell disease. Symptoms & Complications

pfizer.com

Sickle Cell Disease (SCD) Silent Damage

Chapter 22 Mommy and Daughter Talk (Sulcata African Spurred Tortoise)

The Circle of Care Guidebook for Caregivers of Children With Rare and / or Serious illnesses

Source: National Alliance for Caregiving (NAC) Year:2021

There are available resources to help caregivers such as: Caregiver Burnout **Resource** Source: Cleveland Clinic Year:2019, Caregiver Burnout Prevention: Source: Cleveland Clinic Year : 2019

Caregiver Support | oneSCDvoice

https://www.onescdvoice.com

Chapter 23 Sickle Cell Awareness Month (Blue Skies)

National Sickle Cell Awareness month is a great opportunity to be aware of those in your community and those around the world. This article helps you to understand what Sickle Cell Disease is. Throughout the month you can explore research, programs, and the progress of Sickle Cell.

September is National Sickle Cell Awareness Month | NHLBI, NIH Sickle Cell Awareness 2024

sickle cell - NHLBI Search Results

https://www.nhlbi.nih.gov

Sickle Cell Warriors has served as a valuable source of information in the Sickle Cell community and is open to collaborations with other advocacy groups, community-based organizations, Sickle Cell orgs, hospitals, payors, clinics, physicians, universities, research companies, and any who would seed to serve in Sickle Cell disease.

Sickle Cell Warriors is dedicated to providing resources, information, education, research, and support to the Sickle Cell community and healthcare community. Our mission statement can be summarized into five pillars: Education,

Empowerment, Awareness, Research, and Advocacy/Activism. Learn more on the site here **https://sicklecellwarriors.com**

Chapter 24 Breaking New (Guinea Pig)

How much does a bone marrow transplant cost?- Depending on the needs of the patient, the average cost of a bone marrow transplant can range from $80,000 to up to $400,000 before health insurance. helphopelive.org

AABB NEWS CENTER-Bone Marrow Transplant May Be Safe, Cost-Effective Treatment For Sickle Cell Disease March 05,2025

Bone Marrow Transplant May Be Safe, Cost-Effective Treatment for Sickle Cell Disease

Comparative Cost Analysis of Therapy in Sickle Cell Anemia: Supportive Care VS. Bone Marrow Transplant

The sickle cell information center website estimates the cost $150,000 to 250,000. This article explains what it all entails.

Comparative Cost Analysis of Therapy in Sickle Cell Anemia: Supportive Care Vs. Bone Marrow Transplant | Blood | American Society of Hematology

https://doi.org/10.1182/blood.V126.23.4466.4466

Fetal hemoglobin

Fetal hemoglobin-Wikipedia (**https://en.wikipedia.org**)

Structure and genetics, Production, factors affecting oxygen affinity, hereditary persistence of fetal hemoglobin.

Fetal hemoglobin - Wikipedia

Gene Therapy- What is the most important information to know about it.

cost of sickle cell therapy - Search

https://www.casgevy.com/sickle-cell-disease?gclid=c6bbc-36cb3e71ff9626fabed31dbaccd&gclsrc=3p.ds&msclkid=c6bb-c36cb3e71ff9626fabed31dbaccd&utm_source=bing&utm_me-dium=cpc&utm_

campaign=%7CEG%7CDTCB%7CUB%7CSCD%7C-CASG%7CVRX%7CCore%7CBS%20-%20SCD%20Unbrand-ed_Treatment_Exact&utm_term=gene%20treatment%20for%20scd&utm_content=Sickle%20Cell%20Gene%20Treatment%7CTX-T%7CNational%7CA%3A1

htps://www.casgevy.com

Chapter 25 I Don't Remember (Elephant)

Sickle Cell and Memory Problems

3 Comment/Complications of Sickle Cell, Living with Sickle Cell / By SC Warrior

An entry about how you can become sharper and more focused. It also focuses on getting things accomplished at work, school or home.

Sickle Cell and Memory Problems - Sickle Cell Warriors Inc

https://www.sicklecellwarriors.com

Neurocognitive Changes in Sickle Cell Disease: A Comprehensive Review

Chapter 26 (Mena Mother Nature)

Mother Nature- It's important to keep nature in balance because the consequences of upsetting it can be severe. For example, human activities like deforestation, pollution, and global warming are a major threat to the environment.

DON'T MESS WITH MOTHER NATURE-HEAL THE PLANET

There is always a price to pay when humanity disturbs the delicate balance of Mother Nature. Mar 14,2024 Heal the Planet **https://healtheplanet.com**

Over 100 Ways To Heal The Planet — HEAL THE PLANET

Video-Sickle Cell: Natural Selection in Humans/HHMI BioInteractive Video Jan 29, 2024

Hematology - Study of Blood Disorder

Bing Videos

Chapter 27 Happy (Light)

Some Beneficial Lessons from Living With Sickle Cell Disease

What I've learned about resilience, empathy, support, and happiness by Oluwatosin Adesoye/ November 6, 2024

This article brings out that Family, Friends, and Relatives are a great support in helping you to make it through many challenges. Support groups, educating and advocating gives you a purpose in life.

Some beneficial lessons from living with sickle cell disease

sicklecellanemianews.com

History & Timeline of Sickle Cell Disease

Tracing Sickle Cell back to one child, 7,300 years ago 12 March 2018 New research suggests that the history of Sickle Cell disease goes back to a mutation in just one person, a development researchers hope will make treatment less complicated for the many people who suffer from this painful illness. So how have they traced it and why does it matter? The story of Sickle-Cell disease is, first and foremost, a study in how a good thing can come with bad consequences.

Once upon a time in what is now the Sahara Desert, a child was born with heightened immunity to malaria. This defense was important because at the time, this part of Africa was wet and rainy and covered with forest. It was a great habitat for mosquitoes, which carry malaria, a disease that these days kills one child every two minutes. With a better chance against an illness that was a major killer, then as now, this child developed a genetic mutation lived and had children, and those children spread out, all bolstered with extra defenses against malaria and living for longer, and their descendants around the world still have those extra defenses today, more than 250 generations later. *http://bbc.com*

This prolonged battle could be prevented if we go back in history and take the time to read about Sickle Cell Disease. Sickle Cell Disease is caused by inheriting two mutated hemoglobin genes, one from each parent. The mutated gene is sometimes called a Sickle Cell Gene. I hope this book will enlighten my readers by giving them knowledge about what is really in the blood of our culture and what is truly running through our veins.

How do we get Sickle Cell Disease?

Inheritance Sickle Cell conditions are inherited from parents who have the same blood type. It is just like having the same hair color, same color eyes, and other physical traits. It depends on the type of hemoglobin a person has in the red blood cells which depends upon what hemoglobin genes the person inherits from both parents. Therefore, these hemoglobin genes are inherited in two sets. You get one gene from each parent. Let's look at some examples given by the Sickle Cell Association of the National Capital Area.

Examples:

(A) If one parent has Sickle Cell anemia (SS) and the other has normal (AA) blood, all of the children will have sickle cell trait.

(B) If one parent has Sickle Cell anemia (SS) and the other has Sickle Cell anemia (AS), there is a 50% chance (1 chance out of 2) of having a baby with either Sickle Cell disease or Sickle Cell trait with each pregnancy.

(C) When both parents have Sickle Cell trait (AS), they have a 25% chance (1 chance out of 4) of having a baby with Sickle Cell disease with each pregnancy.

(D) If one parent has normal (AA) blood, the other parent has (AS) there is a 50% chance of (1 chance out of 4) of having a baby with Sickle Cell trait or normal (AA)blood.

Researchers also stated that there wasn't just one once upon a time. Instead, several children developed the advantage against malaria separately.

Now for the kicker there were bad consequences about this extra defense against malaria. The fact is if both parents have the gene mutation, their child could end up with Sickle Cell Disease. The consequences are severe pain, shortness of breath, strokes, vision problems and other complications. Some have died at an early age from these complications. The sad fact about it is if both parents inherit the gene, it will not protect people against malaria.

How will you know if you have the trait?

There is a painless blood test that you can take prescribed by your doctor. A laboratory technique which is called Hemoglobin Electrophoresis will determine the type of hemoglobin you have.

There is normal hemoglobin (A), Sickle hemoglobin (S), and other different kinds of hemoglobin like C, D, E, etc. The most common are

Sickle Cell Anemia (SS), Sickle Hemoglobin C Disease (SC), Sickle Beta-Plus Thalassemia and Sickle Beta-Zero Thalassemia. The struggle is real. In my research in authoring this book I didn't even know there was a (HbSO) Sickle-Hemoglobin Sickle Cell Disease. In populations such as Arabian, North African, and Eastern Mediterranean descents have a high frequency of SO disease.

What about Sickle Cell Trait?

People who have the Sickle Cell Trait have more red blood cells than S, therefore they are generally healthy.

Even though Sickle Cell affects many people throughout the world of all backgrounds, the greatest number affected in the U.S. are those with African Ancestry. The Origin Sickle Cell Foundation stated: Sickle Cell Disease is the most common inherited blood disorder in the United States and is estimated to affect more than 100,00 Americans. Every year, more than 2,000 babies are born with this disease. Worldwide, it is estimated that over 300,000 babies are born with Sickle Cell disease every single year. The origin of the mutation that led to Sickle-Cell Gene derives from at least four independent mutational events, three in Africa and a fourth in either Saudi Arabia or central India. African medical literature reports elements of this disease tracking back to 1670 in one Ghanaian family. These independent events occurred between 3,000 and 6,000 generations ago. Approximately 70-150,000 years ago. Research shows that the mutation causing Sickle Cell Disease arose in Africa thousands of years ago to help protect against malaria." It had various names in Africa. It depended on the tribal languages. Let me tell you a little story that traces Sickle Cell back to one child, 7,300 years ago. New research by BBC suggests that the history of Sickle Cell disease goes back to a mutation in just one person. They stated the story of Sickle Cell Disease is, first and foremost, a study in how a good thing can come with bad consequences.

Researchers also stated that there wasn't just one once upon a time. Instead, several children developed the advantage against malaria separately.

Now for the kicker. There were bad consequences about this extra defense against malaria. The fact is if both parents have the gene mutation, their child could end up with Sickle Cell Disease. The consequences are severe pain, shortness of breath, strokes, vision problems and other complications. Some have died at an early age from these complications. The sad fact about it is if both parents inherit the gene, it will not protect people against malaria. https://www.sicklecellmn.org

What are the types of Sickle Cell Disease?

Hemoglobin is the protein in red blood cells that carries oxygen. It normally has two alpha chains and two beta chains.

Four main types of Sickle Cell Anemia caused by different mutations in genes

1. Hemoglobin SS disease
2. Hemoglobin SC disease
3. Hemoglobin SB+(beta)thalassemia
4. Hemoglobin SB O (Beta-zero)
5. Hemoglobin SD, Hemoglobin SE, and Hemoglobin SO more rare and usually don't have severe symptoms

www.Healthline.com

(National Heart, Lung, and Blood Institute) – Visit this site to see the timeline 1910-2010. Sickle Cell Disease: Research, Programs, and Progress-Sickle Cell Disease) www.nhlbi.nih.gov

Can Sickle Cell be stopped?

Sickle Cell anemia is an inherited blood disorder. Because it's a genetic condition someone is born with, there is no way to prevent the disease, so scientists are constantly investigating ways that the disease can be stopped before it passes to the next generation.

Is there a cure for Sickle Cell Disease? Is there a cure coming soon for Sickle Cell?

In December 2023, the U.S. Food and Drug Administration approved two new gene therapies that are transformative therapies for Sickle Cell Disease.

One treatment adds a modified gene into the body and the other treatment makes a change to a gene that is already in the body. NIH (National Heart, Lung, and Blood Institute Article

(1)Exagamglogene autotemcel (Suspension (liquid) to be injected intravenously (into a vein) by a doctor or nurse in a hospital or infusion center) is in a class of medications called autologous cellular immunotherapy, a type of medication prepared using cells from the patient's own blood. It is used in adults and children 12 years of age and older. It works by helping the body to make hemoglobin which helps keep cells from sickling in SCD and helps produce more healthy hemoglobin in TDT patients. Brand name Casgevy. Medlineplus.gov

(2) Lovotibeglogene autotemcel (Suspension (liquid) to be injected intravenously (into a vein) by a doctor or nurse in a hospital or infusion center) makes changes to a gene that is already in the body. It is used in adults and children 12 years of age and older. Lovotibeglogene is in a class of medications called autologous cellular immunotherapy, a type of medication prepared using cells from the patient's own blood. It works by helping the body to start producing normal red blood cells. Brand names Lyfgenia. Medlineplus.gov

https://www.nhlbi.nih.gov.>health

Who needs a Sickle Cell Test?

Newborns are regularly screened for SCD soon after birth. Early diagnosis is the key.

Other people who should get tested include:

- Immigrants who haven't been tested in their home countries
- Children who move from one state to another and haven't been tested
- Anyone displaying symptoms of the disease

http://www.healthline.com

Timeline

DID YOU KNOW?

SICKLE CELL WAS THE FIRST DIAGNOSED GENETIC DISEASE, AND THE FIRST TO BE LINKED TO THE HEMOGLOBIN PROTEIN

Sickle Cell Over the Years

- **1910-** Dr. James Herrick notes the sickle shape of red blood cells, identifying **sickle cell anemia**
- **1949-**Sickle cell identified as a **genetic disease**
- **1972-** **The National Association for Sickle Cell Disease** is established
- **1972-** **National Sickle Cell Anemia Control Act** is signed into law establishing education, information, screening, testing, counseling, research, and treatment programs for sickle cell
- **1994-**Long-term blood transfusions are found to **decrease hospitalizations**
- **1998-First treatment for sickle cell is approved** by the US Food and Drug Administration (FDA)
- **2006-**The World Health Organization recognizes sickle cell as a global health crisis; **the United States implements mandatory newborn screenings in every state**
- **Blood stem cell transplants** are shown to stop progression in sickle cell
- **2017-FDA approves second treatment for sickle cell** after 19 years

- **2018-The Sickle Cell Disease and Other Heritable Blood Disorders Research Disease and Other Heritable Blood Disorders Research, Surveillance, Prevention, and Treatment Act** is signed into law
- **2019- FDA approves two new drugs** to reduce pain crises and treat sickle cell
- **2023-FDA approves first two gene therapies** to treat sickle cell disease

Understanding Sickle Cell- https://sparksicklecellchange.com

About the author

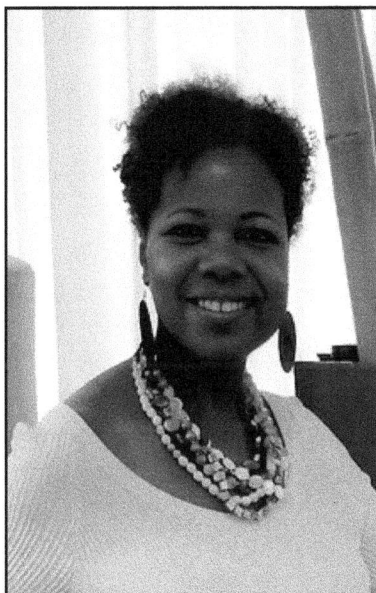

Iris Wright-Hart grew up on the Eastern Shore of Maryland, where she lives with her devoted husband, Jeffrey Hart. For over 45 years, she has been a loving wife and dedicated mother of four, taking great pride in her six grandchildren, her work as an early childhood educator, and her active ministry as one of Jehovah's Witnesses. A standout memory—winning the 200-meter hurdles at the 1977 Maryland State Championship—still fuels the passion she brings to her work and relationships today. Like the iris flower for which she is named, Iris symbolizes faith, courage, hope, and wisdom—qualities she strives to embody and share, especially with Sickle Cell Warriors.

www.ingramcontent.com/pod-product-compliance
Lightning Source LLC
Chambersburg PA
CBHW052017030426
42335CB00026B/3178

9 781967 082506